Innovations for Urban Sanitation

Praise for this book

'The urban sanitation sector suffers from a lack of effective engagement with the people who will use the services. Developments are usually driven by engineers, technology and regulations, with little heed paid to the capacities, aspirations, motivations and affordability of the sanitation services to the user. *Innovations for Urban Sanitation: Adapting community-led approaches* contributes to redressing that balance and giving voice to the community and sanitation users. This useful new book applies what has been learned from using participatory tools in rural and urban sanitation to provide practical approaches to partner better with communities in urban sanitation projects – big and small. As a workbook it provides a menu of tools and techniques to mix and match for different types of urban sanitation project. Projects and programmes which systematically use these approaches will achieve better community engagement and increased ownership and thus improve the sustainability and outcomes of urban sanitation investments.'

Isabel Blackett, Consultant, Inclusive Sanitation in Practice (ISP)

'A timely and valuable book for anyone wanting to better understand the complexities of CLTS in urban settings. The authors helpfully combine comprehensive descriptions, practical guidance and tools for integrating CLTS into sustainable urban sanitation services.'

Rebecca Scott, Lecturer in Public Health Engineering,
WEDC, Loughborough University, UK

Innovations for Urban Sanitation
Adapting Community-led Approaches

Jamie Myers, Sue Cavill, Samuel Musyoki,
Katherine Pasteur and Lucy Stevens

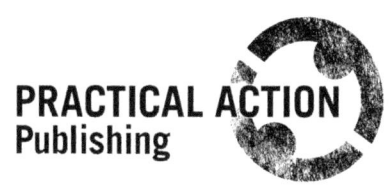

Practical Action Publishing
Rugby, Warwickshire, UK
www.practicalactionpublishing.org

© Institute of Development Studies, CLTS Knowledge Hub (2018)

The moral right of the authors to be identified as editors of the work and the contributors to be identified as contributors of this work have been asserted under sections 77 and 78 of the Copyright Designs and Patents Act 1988.

This open access article is distributed under a Creative Commons Attribution Non-commercial No-derivatives CC BY-NC-ND license. This allows the reader to copy and redistribute the material; but appropriate credit must be given, the material must not be used for commercial purposes, and if the material is transformed or built upon the modified material may not be distributed. For further information see https://creativecommons.org/licenses/by-nc-nd/4.0/legalcode

Product or corporate names may be trademarks or registered trademarks, and are used only for identification and explanation without intent to infringe.

A catalogue record for this book is available from the British Library.

A catalogue record for this book has been requested from the Library of Congress.

ISBN 978-1-78853-017-0 Paperback
ISBN 978-1-78853-016-3 Hardback
ISBN 978-1-78044-736-0 Library Pdf
ISBN 978-1-78044-738-4 ePub

Citation: Myers, J. Cavill, S. Musyoki, S. Pasteur, K. Stevens, L. (2018) *Innovations for Urban Sanitation: Adapting Community-led Approaches*, Rugby, UK, Practical Action Publishing, <http://dx.doi.org/10.3362/9781780447360>

Since 1974, Practical Action Publishing has published and disseminated books and information in support of international development work throughout the world. Practical Action Publishing is a trading name of Practical Action Publishing Ltd (Company Reg. No. 1159018), the wholly owned publishing company of Practical Action. Practical Action Publishing trades only in support of its parent charity objectives and any profits are covenanted back to Practical Action (Charity Reg. No. 247257, Group VAT Registration No. 880 9924 76).

The views and opinions in this publication are those of the author and do not represent those of Practical Action Publishing Ltd or its parent charity Practical Action. Reasonable efforts have been made to publish reliable data and information, but the authors and publisher cannot assume responsibility for the validity of all materials or for the consequences of their use.

This document/book has been financed by the Swedish International Development Cooperation Agency, Sida. Sida does not necessarily share the views expressed in this material. Responsibility for its contents rests entirely with the author.

Cover illustration by Jamie Eke
Cover design by: RCO.design
Printed in the United Kingdom

Contents

Tables, boxes, and figures	vii
Author and organization biographies	xi
Acronyms and abbreviations	xii
Glossary of key terms	xiii
Overview	xv
Acknowledgements	xvi

Chapter 1: Introduction	**1**
Who is this guide for?	3
The principles of U-CLTS	3
Comparing the use of CLTS in urban versus rural settings	4
U-CLTS across urban typologies	7
Challenges for U-CLTS	12
Roles and responsibilities within U-CLTS	14
How to use this guide	16
Dos and don'ts	18
Notes for users	20

PART 1: The guide

Chapter 2: Stage 1: Assessment and preparation (pre-triggering)	**23**
Purpose of assessment and preparation	24
Situation analysis	27
Stakeholder analysis and identifying key partners	31
Key partner capacity building and selection of communities	37
Preparing to enter the community	38
Dos and don'ts for assessment and preparation (pre-triggering)	39
Notes for users	41
Chapter 3: Stage 2: U-CLTS triggering and institutional advocacy	**43**
Purpose of U-CLTS triggering	43
Community triggering	45
Community-led action planning processes	59
Institutional advocacy and action planning	63
Institutional advocacy tools and tactics	65
Dos and don'ts for triggering, advocacy, and action planning	70
Notes for users	72

http://dx.doi.org/10.3362/9781780447360.000

Chapter 4: Stage 3: Integrating U-CLTS across the sanitation chain — 75
Purpose of integrating U-CLTS across the sanitation chain — 75
Revising and enforcing regulations across the sanitation chain — 78
Safe capture and containment — 79
Safe emptying and transportation — 90
Safe treatment, disposal, and possible reuse — 92
Associated waste streams — 93
Dos and don'ts for integrating U-CLTS across the sanitation chain — 96
Notes for users — 97

Chapter 5: Stage 4: Maintaining momentum — 99
Purpose of maintaining momentum — 99
Follow-up — 101
Monitoring — 105
Verification, certification, and celebration — 110
Sustainability — 112
Dos and don'ts and action points for maintaining momentum — 114
Notes for users — 116

PART 2: Case studies

Chapter 6: U-CLTS case studies — 121
Case Study 1: Choma, Zambia — 121
Case Study 2: Eight towns in Ethiopia — 125
Case Study 3: Fort Dauphin, Madagascar — 127
Case Study 4: Gulariya, Nepal — 130
Case Study 5: Hawassa, Ethiopia — 133
Case Study 6: Himbirti, Eritrea — 135
Case Study 7: Iringa, Tanzania — 139
Case Study 8: IUWASH, Indonesia — 141
Case Study 9: Kabwe, Zambia — 145
Case Study 10: Logo, Nigeria — 147
Case Study 11: Mathare 10, Nairobi, Kenya — 149
Case Study 12: Nakuru, Kenya — 153
Case Study 13: New Delhi, India — 157
Case Study 14: Ribaué and Rapale, Mozambique — 159
Case Study 15: Small towns in Northern and Southern Nigeria — 162

Conclusion — 165
References — 167

Tables, boxes, and figures

Tables

1.1	SDG sanitation and sanitation-related targets	2
1.2	Rural OD versus faecal waste risks in urban areas	5
1.3	Some practical challenges of U-CLTS implementation	13
1.4	Challenges and opportunities for using a U-CLTS approach	14
1.5	Roles and responsibilities of different sanitation stakeholders	15
1.6	Tools and tactics listed under each stage	17
1.7	General dos and don'ts for U-CLTS	18
2.1	Dos and don'ts: assessment and preparation	39
3.1	Actions likely to be needed by each stakeholder group	63
3.2	Dos and don'ts: triggering, advocacy, and action planning	70
4.1	Dos and don'ts: integrating U-CLTS across the sanitation chain	96
5.1	Dos and don'ts: maintaining momentum	114

Boxes

1.1	Rural sanitation and CLTS	4
1.2	Guide to boxes	18
2.1	Implications of vulnerability for U-CLTS	26
2.2	Political economy analysis for faecal sludge management	35
3.1	Guides for urban sanitation planning	62

Figures

1.1	The urban sanitation value chain	4
1.2	Examples of faecal pollution routes in urban environments	5
1.3	Characteristics of different urban typologies and the associated U-CLTS case study	8
2.1	Clusters of disadvantage	26
2.2	Potential key social influencers	36
3.1	Faecal waste or shit flow diagram	67
4.1	Actions along the sanitation chain	77
5.1	Billboard promoting handwashing at key times, Gulariya, Nepal	103
5.2	Hoarding board in rural town of Shebedion, Ethiopia	113

Tools

2.1	Baseline survey	29
2.2	Participatory household enumeration survey	30
2.3	Venn diagram mapping	32
2.4	Political economy analysis	33
2.5	Social network mapping	35
3.1	Sanitation street theatre	47
3.2	Sanitation mapping	50
3.3	Shit calculation	52
3.4	Household medical expenses calculation	53
3.5	Transect walk	54
3.6	Shit and water	55
3.7	Faecal–oral contamination routes	55
3.8	Participatory video/photography	56
3.9	Analysing water contamination	57
3.10	Scenario planning	61
3.11	Ranking and prioritization tool	62
3.12	City Sanitation Plans or Sanitation Master Plans	63
3.13	Faecal waste/shit flow diagrams	65
3.14	Exposure visits	68
3.15	Sharing the numbers	68
3.16	Landlord forums	69
4.1	Participatory technology development	83
4.2	Participatory tools for socially inclusive design	83
4.3	Participatory analysis of market systems for sanitation	85
4.4	Supply chain analysis	86
4.5	Solid waste calculations	94
5.1	Community exchange visits	102
5.2	Visual monitoring	106
5.3	Institutional performance scoring	107
5.4	Community scorecards	107
5.5	Intercommunity monitoring	108
5.6	Mobile phone monitoring	109
5.7	Celebrating progress	112
5.8	Hoarding boards	112

Tactics

3.1	Triggering homogeneous groups	47
3.2	Mob triggering	48
3.3	Plot/compound triggering	49
3.4	Sharing community triggering with key stakeholders	67
5.1	Sanitation ambassadors	101
5.2	Use of traditional and social media	102
5.3	Women's groups	104

Examples

2.1	Considering vulnerability and planning for safety	27
2.2	Baseline data collection	29
2.3	Enumeration surveys	31
2.4	Influencers from different U-CLTS programmes	37
2.5	Key partners	38
3.1	Triggering homogeneous groups	48
3.2	Mob triggering	48
3.3	Compound triggering	49
3.4	GIS mapping	52
3.5	Triggering for connecting to existing infrastructure	57
3.6	Using water contamination data	58
3.7	Multiple stakeholder planning event	65
4.1	enforcing and revising regulation	78
4.2	Community actions	82
4.3	Assessing market barriers	85
4.4	Improving access to finance	88
4.5	Community-managed facilities	89
4.6	Community involvement in FSM	91
4.7	Capacity development for FSM	92
4.8	Container-based sanitation	93
4.9	Waste collection and income generation	95
5.1	Engaging women's groups	104
5.2	Community-based monitoring	106
5.3	Using apps to monitor progress	110
5.4	Encouraging competition between local bodies: Swachh Survekshan	111
5.5	Kick-starting a social movement	114

Tips

2.1	Consider vulnerability	25
3.1	Triggering for what?	50
3.2	Considering vulnerability	50
3.3	Transect walks	55
4.1	Right to sanitation and vulnerable groups	89

Author and organization biographies

Jamie Myers – Research Officer based at the Institute of Development Studies, looking at the use of CLTS and other similar community-based participatory processes in rural, peri-urban and urban environments.

Sue Cavill – Freelance consultant with over 17 years of experience in the WASH sector, from implementing programmes to policy research and analysis.

Samuel Musyoki – Country Director, Plan International Zambia with a background in anthropology and over 18 years experience as a trainer in participatory development processes.

Katherine Pasteur – Freelance consultant working alongside The CLTS Knowledge Hub, The CLTS Foundation, and NGOs such as Practical Action to document the evolving experiences and lessons from CLTS practice around the world.

Lucy Stevens – Policy & Practice Adviser at Practical Action with 10 years of experience leading learning initiatives in urban WASH and waste management.

Institute of Development Studies (IDS) is a leading global institution for development research, teaching and learning, and impact and communications, based at the University of Sussex. IDS have been working in support of CLTS for over a decade. During this time CLTS has become an international movement.

Plan International is a development and humanitarian organization that advances children's rights and equality for girls. They use the CLTS approach in countries across Africa and Asia and in peri-urban and urban areas in Ethiopia, India, Kenya, and Zambia.

Practical Action is an international NGO that uses technology to challenge poverty in development countries. They promote the CLTS approach with partners and local governments, demonstrating best practice and developing innovative technologies for clean water and waste management, and they work with national and city governments to ensure that poor people are included in sanitation planning.

Acronyms and abbreviations

CBE	Community-based entrepreneur
CBO	Community-based organization
CLTS	Community-Led Total Sanitation
CLUES	Community-Led Urban Environmental Sanitation
CSO	Civil society organisation
FCHV	Female Community Health Volunteer
FSM	Faecal sludge management
GIS	Geographic information systems
GPS	Global positioning system
LGA	Local government area
NGO	Non-governmental organization
OD	Open defecation
ODF	Open defecation free
PTD	Participatory technology development
SDG	Sustainable Development Goal
SME	Small- and medium-sized enterprise
U-CLTS	Urban Community-Led Total Sanitation
UN	United Nations
VIP	Ventilated improved pit
WASH	Water, sanitation, and hygiene
WatSan	Water and sanitation

Glossary of key terms

Key terms	Definition
Community-Led Total Sanitation (CLTS)	A methodology for mobilizing communities to completely eliminate open defecation (OD). Communities are facilitated to conduct their own appraisal and analysis of OD and take their own action to become ODF (open defecation free).
Enabling environment	A range of components needed to support the delivery of sustained sanitation services. These include policy, institutional frameworks, financing, capacity, and regulations.
Faecal sludge	Raw or partially digested slurry or semi-solid waste, consisting of excreta and black water, with or without grey water. Faecal sludge may be contained in many ways: for example, pit latrines, unsewered public toilets, septic tanks, aqua privies, and dry toilets. Faecal sludge is highly variable in consistency, quantity, and concentration.
Faecal sludge management (FSM)	The storage, collection, transport, treatment, and safe end use or disposal of faecal sludge.
Fixed-point open defecation	The use of an unimproved latrine where excreta remains exposed to the environment and continues to be a public health risk: for example, the latrine is overflowing, there is no slab, or people are defecating on the slab.
Flying toilet	A bag or carton used to defecate in which is then thrown away or dumped in the surrounding environment.
Human right to sanitation	Explicit recognition by the UN General Assembly in 2010: 'the right to safe and clean drinking water and sanitation [is] a human right that is essential for the full enjoyment of life and all human rights' (Resolution 64/292, 1, UN Doc. A/RES/64/292, 3 August 2010).
Improved sanitation	A facility that hygienically separate faeces from human contact.
Open defecation	The practice of defecating outside in the open, often in public spaces.

xiv GLOSSARY OF KEY TERMS

People who are marginalized	A person who is outside the main body of society or has limited decision-making power within it. Such people may have limited resources (financial or otherwise) and they do not automatically gain the same benefits from programmes as others. They have often faced historical or cultural discrimination and are under-represented in political decision-making (House et al., 2014).
People who are vulnerable	A person is more vulnerable in any given context when they are less able/unable to cope with problems or hazards and hence are more at risk. They are likely to have limited influence and control over decisions or resources (House et al., 2014).
People who have special circumstances	A person who has special circumstances is considered for the purposes of this toolkit to have needs that may not be met by services or responses that do not consider people's different needs (for example, accessibility for people with limited mobility). They may or may not also be vulnerable or marginalized (House et al., 2014).
Safely managed sanitation	The use of a private improved sanitation facility that is not shared with other households and where excreta is safely disposed in situ or is transported and treated off-site, and where there is also a handwashing facility with soap and water. Improved sanitation facilities include flush/pour flush to a piped sewer, septic tank, or pit latrine, composting toilet, or pit latrine with a slab.
Sanitation chain	The process by which sanitation waste is contained, emptied, transported, treated, and disposed/reused safely so that it does not come into contact with people or contaminate the local environment.
Shit-free environment	An urban environment where all excreta is safely managed, where all have access to affordable sanitation and related services, and where faecal matter is not entering from other communities or being transferred from one community to another.
Solid waste management	The collection, treatment, and disposal of solid material that is discarded because it has served its purpose or is no longer useful.
Urban Community-Led Total Sanitation (U-CLTS)	A process towards building the commitment of individuals, groups, and institutions to take individual and collective action to achieve safely managed sanitation for all in urban communities. It requires combined individual, community, and institutional action to achieve this.

Overview

This guide has been developed in response to calls from practitioners for support in using CLTS approaches in urban settings – which is referred to throughout as Urban Community-Led Total Sanitation (U-CLTS). Although CLTS is already being implemented in urban settings, practitioners highlight a lack of clarity on many of the possible practical steps involved. This book hopes to fill this gap. It also aims to increase awareness among urban WASH professionals of the potential of U-CLTS to improve different parts of the sanitation chain. In particular, the authors wish to encourage practitioners to recognize the capacity of communities to make sanitation safer and more effective.

Part 1 includes an introduction and overview of U-CLTS approaches. It is intended to improve the reader's knowledge of the added value of this approach to existing urban sanitation approaches. It provides suggestions on how to design a U-CLTS programme or use U-CLTS techniques and tools as part of broader sanitation programmes. It offers a number of tools for implementers and regulators of urban sanitation programmes. The focus in this section is on what is needed, what to do, why, and how to do it.

Part 2 describes a number of case studies. The focus is on how others have done it. The cases presented provide additional inspiration and ideas and are not to be copied and pasted. Experiences are drawn from Ethiopia, Eritrea, India, Indonesia, Kenya, Mozambique, Madagascar, Nepal, Nigeria, Tanzania and Zambia. We expect this section to expand as more cases are documented. Readers are encouraged to send additional case studies to CLTS@ids.ac.uk. New experiences will be uploaded to http://www.communityledtotalsanitation.org/Innovations-for-Urban-Sanitation-casestudies.

This document has been developed by the CLTS Knowledge Hub, Practical Action, and Plan International with contributions from a wide range of actors. It has been funded by Sida and has been co-published by a number of organizations. For further information please contact: the CLTS Knowledge Hub at CLTS@ids.ac.uk.

Acknowledgements

This book has been a collaborative effort between the Institute of Development Studies, Plan International and Practical Action. It came about following a workshop held in Addis Ababa in June 2016 which explored the use of CLTS in peri-urban and urban environments. Thanks are needed for all the participants who collectively developed the foundations of this guide. In addition, we would like to thank the following people for their support throughout the process.

We are indebted to the case study authors whose rich experiences and innovative thinking are demonstrated throughout Part 2, and also to others whose work we draw on.

We would like to thank Petra Bongartz, Stacey Townsend, Naomi Vernon, and Robert Chambers of the CLTS Knowledge Hub who have read drafts, edited, given ideas, and supported the process throughout.

We are grateful to Isabel Blackett, who, due to her commitment to see more participatory and empowering approaches, has spent a considerable amount of time reviewing the text and sharing her knowledge and experience of the complexity of inclusive urban sanitation. We also thank the peer reviewers Christoph Lüthi, Georges Mikhael, Diane Mitlin, and Rebecca Scott, whose productive comments helped strengthen the guide.

Furthermore, we are grateful to the staff of Tilton House where the writing team spent a week developing an initial draft, to Clare Tawney and Practical Action for their support getting our text from Microsoft Word to the guide you currently have in your hands (or on your computer screen), and to Jamie Eke for his illustrations.

We would also like to thank the Swedish International Development Cooperation Agency (Sida) and the CLTS Knowledge Hub Programme Manager Johan Sundberg for the support they have given the Hub since 2014.

CHAPTER 1
Introduction

Abstract

Three out of 10 people in urban areas do not use improved sanitation facilities, and one out of 10 people are forced to practise open defecation. Still higher proportions do not have access to safely managed sanitation facilities, where the faecal sludge is contained and either left in situ or safely emptied, transported, and delivered to a treatment plant. Urban Community-Led Total Sanitation (U-CLTS) is a process that can contribute to building commitment of individuals, groups, and institutions to take individual and collective action to achieve safely managed sanitation for all in urban communities. This opening chapter provides an introduction to U-CLTS and has been designed to show readers how CLTS can be adapted for urban environments. It gives an overview of the approach and explains its principles. It focuses on what U-CLTS can offer across different urban typologies, how and why it needs to be adapted to tackle the sanitation service chain, and the challenges participatory, community-led approaches are likely to face.

Keywords: Urban Community-Led Total Sanitation, sanitation service chain, faecal sludge management, safely managed sanitation, equity and inclusion, Sustainable Development Goals

Over half the world's population now live in urban areas. While 83 per cent of the global urban population uses a basic sanitation facility (WHO and UNICEF, 2017), three out of 10 people in urban areas do not use improved sanitation facilities, and one out of 10 people still practise open defecation (OD) (WHO and UNICEF, 2016). Faecal sludge management (FSM) is less well monitored at present, but recent global estimates suggest that only 43 per cent of urban dwellers can rely on a safely managed sanitation facility (WHO and UNICEF, 2017), where the faecal sludge is contained and either left in situ or safely emptied, transported, and delivered to a treatment plant. On-site sanitation is reported to be the main form of improved sanitation in the urban areas of Central Asia and Southern Asia, Oceania and sub-Saharan Africa, but only 13 per cent of these systems are estimated to be safely managed (WHO and UNICEF, 2017). This lack of safely managed sanitation and the density of settlement often lead to health indicators that are worse than for rural areas

http://dx.doi.org/10.3362/9781780447360.001

(in terms of prevalence of diarrhoeal diseases, deaths of children under five, and rates of malnutrition and stunting associated with poor sanitation).

Sustainable Development Goal (SDG) 6 recognizes that a range of different methods, tools, and approaches will be needed to reach the targets for universal access to sanitation. SDG 6.B explicitly recognizes the need to strengthen the participation of local communities in improving water and sanitation management. However, participation and community-led actions do not mean that governments, institutions, and service providers do not need to be responsible and accountable. Increasing community participation in planning and management for urban sanitation can improve the effectiveness and equity of these services, as has been demonstrated with the Community-Led Urban Environmental Sanitation approach (Lüthi et al., 2011).

Urban Community-Led Total Sanitation (U-CLTS) is a process that can contribute to building the commitment of individuals, groups, and institutions to take individual and collective action to achieve safely managed sanitation for all in urban communities. It requires combined individual, community, and institutional action to achieve this. Although not a complete solution by itself, it is an important piece of a larger puzzle. It offers a set of approaches, tools, and tactics that are available to practitioners to ensure safely managed sanitation. The U-CLTS approach has the potential to contribute not just to SDG 6 but also to SDG 11 on cities, and to SDGs targeting the reduction of inequalities and the promotion of inclusive societies (see Table 1.1). As a pro-poor development strategy, U-CLTS can mobilize poor urban communities to collectively take their own actions and work with other stakeholders to provide safely managed sanitation, hygiene, and water services and ensure no one is left behind.

Table 1.1 SDG sanitation and sanitation-related targets

6.2 By 2030, achieve access to adequate and equitable sanitation and hygiene for all and end open defecation, paying special attention to the needs of women and girls and those in vulnerable situations.
6.3 By 2030, improve water quality by reducing pollution, eliminating dumping and minimizing release of hazardous chemicals and materials, halving the proportion of untreated wastewater and substantially increasing recycling and safe reuse globally.
6.B Support and strengthen the participation of local communities in improving water and sanitation management.
11.1 By 2030, ensure access for all to adequate, safe, and affordable housing and basic services and upgrade slums.
11.3 By 2030, enhance inclusive and sustainable urbanization and capacity for participatory, integrated, and sustainable human settlement planning and management in all countries.
11.6 By 2030, reduce the adverse per capita environmental impact of cities, including by paying special attention to air quality and municipal and other waste management.

This guide aims to contribute to current thinking and practice in U-CLTS, drawing on examples of how it has been applied and the successes and challenges it has encountered thus far.

Who is this guide for?

This guide is predominantly designed for those working in government, in international and local non-governmental organizations (NGOs), and in bilateral and multilateral agencies wanting to increase citizen participation and facilitate community-led partnerships to improve sanitation in peri-urban and urban settings. Furthermore, it is for CLTS facilitators more used to working in rural areas and unsure how to work in towns and cities, as well as for urban sanitation professionals wanting to learn more about what U-CLTS can offer for a shit-free environment in an urban context.

The principles of U-CLTS

The focus on a set of core aims is what defines U-CLTS. While many of these principles may appear to be a common-sense approach to any sanitation intervention, they are not yet systematically tested and applied. They include the following:

- *Participation and empowerment.* Community members are at the heart of the process and drive the agenda, taking a central role in advocacy and decision-making. They are supported to take actions where possible and catalyse advocacy efforts to solve their sanitation challenges and work with others to achieve their rights to services.
- *Collective behaviour change and collective action.* This requires the process to focus on all. Everyone must change unsafe sanitation practices in order for the risk of faecal contamination to be eliminated.
- *Community ownership.* A community-led process cannot respond to all sanitation and hygiene needs across the sanitation chain (see Figure 1.1) in urban areas. However, ownership is still possible through communities taking their own actions and can also be built symbolically through the community participating in decision-making processes along with other stakeholders.
- *Demand creation through triggering.* The use of tools that evoke powerful emotions, usually disgust, enable the entire community to confront the negative impacts of OD, bad FSM, and poor sanitation. The tools aim to get institutional and community-level agreements and action, recognizing that by working together the quality of sanitation can be improved.
- *Natural Leaders.* Community-based agents of change or champions should emerge through the U-CLTS process and help lead and support subsequent activities.
- *Total sanitation.* U-CLTS is not considered successful unless everyone is using appropriate safely managed sanitation facilities that are sustained

4 INNOVATIONS FOR URBAN SANITATION

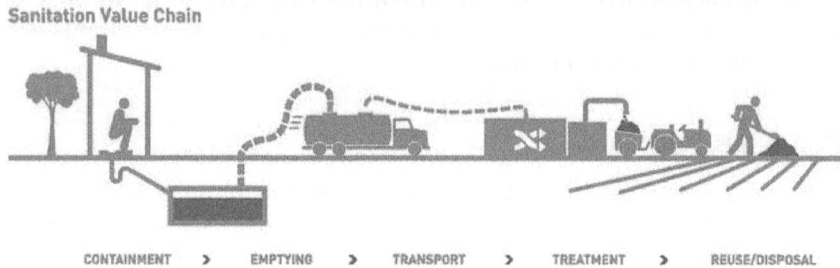

Figure 1.1 The urban sanitation value chain
Source: BMGF, 2015.

over time. The aim is a local and broader environment free of all faecal waste rather than just an open defecation-free (ODF) community, and this requires attention to adequate provision, maintenance of facilities, and faecal waste service provision. Consequently, actions will be needed by different actors across the sanitation chain (see Figure 1.1).

U-CLTS is not designed to take responsibilities away from government and service providers, but in many cases it will support and encourage them and will sometimes also hold them to account.

Comparing the use of CLTS in urban versus rural settings

OD in urban areas is often driven more by necessity than preference: space constraints, insecurity of housing or land tenure, high housing and population density, illegal settlements, living in challenging environments, inability to get an existing latrine emptied, and poor landlord–tenant relationships are all factors that drive OD. However – and more importantly – people are exposed to faeces due to a wider number of reasons in urban areas (see Table 1.2 and Figure 1.2) beyond just OD, which is relatively low compared with rural areas.

Box 1.1 Rural sanitation and CLTS

Community-Led Total Sanitation (CLTS) was pioneered by Dr Kamal Kar together with the Village Education Resource Centre in rural Bangladesh. Communities are facilitated to conduct their own appraisal and analysis of the sanitation context and take their own action to make their community open defecation free (ODF).

The approach has since spread across Africa, Asia and Latin America. In rural areas it is concerned with tackling OD and getting communities to work together to build individual household toilets. The successful outcome of any CLTS intervention is an ODF community.

Sources: Kar with Chambers, 2008; http://www.communityledtotalsanitation.org/page/clts-approach

---

INTRODUCTION 5

Table 1.2 Rural OD versus faecal waste risks in urban areas

Rural	Urban
OD means open exposure to faeces from:	Environment contaminated by shit (or faecal waste). Open exposure to faeces from:
• Almost all from OD. • Some fixed-point OD due to the use of unimproved poor-quality toilets.	• Fixed-point OD from direct toilet discharge and poor-quality toilets and around dysfunctional, blocked, or full latrine pits and septic tanks. • OD in 'hotspots' – typically open spaces, river banks, seashores, and private spaces. • Hanging toilets directly over drains, rivers, ponds, lakes, and canals. • Flying toilets (excreta in plastic bags thrown away). • Pits and septic tanks allowed to overflow into drains and water bodies. • Faecal sludge dumped nearby or unsafely elsewhere, after toilets have been emptied. • Faecal sludge entering neighbourhoods from outside, including through dysfunctional sewerage systems, drainage, flooding, dumping, etc.

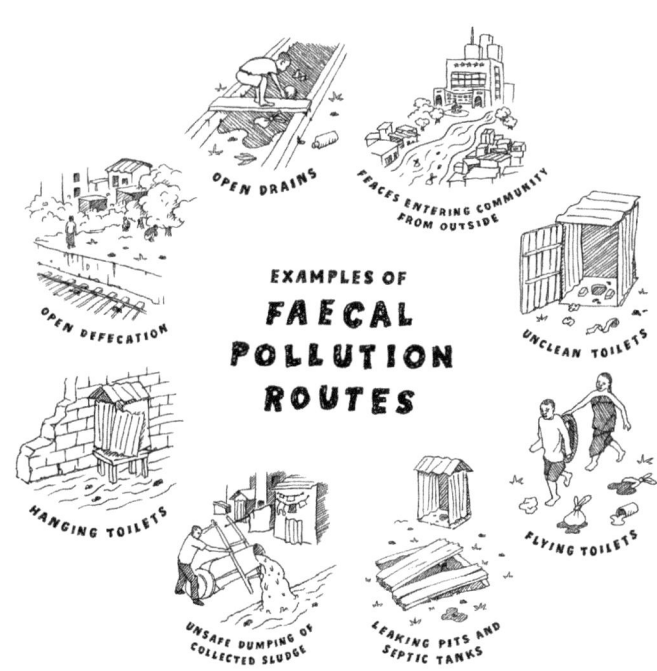

Figure 1.2 Examples of faecal pollution routes in urban environments
Source: CLTS Knowledge Hub. Illustration by Jamie Eke.

Furthermore, exposure to faecal matter occurs due to breakdowns across the sanitation service chain (Figure 1.1). This includes not only the containment of faecal sludge but also storage, emptying, transport, treatment, and disposal/reuse. Therefore, attention needs to be paid to services, service providers, and broader urban development plans, all of which will involve a greater number of stakeholders.

Consequently, a successful outcome in an urban context is a completely shit-free environment rather than just an ODF community; this requires attention to adequate provision, maintenance of sanitation facilities, and faecal sludge service provision. A shit-free environment requires:

- everyone using a safely managed sanitation facility which is connected to a safe and appropriate FSM chain;
- affordable sanitation services that are available for all sectors of the population, irrespective of where they live and work;
- facilities and services that are communal or shared between households when private household facilities are not possible, and that are culturally acceptable;
- if shared or community toilets are most appropriate, they must be affordable, accessible, well maintained, and shared between a minimal number of users;
- public toilets available for use in all public places such as markets, transport hubs, and public buildings;
- clean and safe toilets in schools, clinics, and other institutions used by the public and workers;
- shit produced elsewhere not entering communities or being transferred from one community to another.

Similar to the ODF outcome in a rural context, a shit-free environment is not the end point but an important milestone.

Actions required therefore extend beyond building individual household toilets to the different stages along the sanitation chain. These may include: appropriate operation and maintenance of community toilets; cleaning of communal areas; paying for FSM services; and the use of communal toilets or connections to existing infrastructure, such as sewerage networks. Behaviour change does not relate exclusively to changing individual behaviours but also involves collectively advocating for access to safe services from service providers and government.

Urban sanitation services include a wide array of stakeholders and institutions, and often there is duplication, gaps, and a lack of clarity about which actors are responsible for different parts of the sanitation chain. Furthermore, there is often a lack of coordination between stakeholders and a tendency to focus on infrastructure-based solutions. There may be low political prioritization to tackle sanitation or to incorporate community-based initiatives and/or weak capacity. However, their involvement in triggering and maintaining a shit-free environment will be essential.

U-CLTS does not necessarily mean following processes and tools that have proved successful in rural communities across the world, but rather using similar principles and working with stakeholders to collectively design an intervention for a specific town or city. It will mean working as part of, or in the context of, a broader government or development partner sanitation programme.

U-CLTS across urban typologies

The term 'urban' refers to the characteristics of a town or city, and these vary from place to place. Typical features could include access to infrastructure and services; commercial, education, and government centres; and high population densities in some areas. U-CLTS has been applied in a range of projects and programmes across the spectrum from rural to urban, from small rural towns in Gulariya, Nepal, to a densely populated slum in Mathare 10, Nairobi, Kenya, as illustrated in Figure 1.3. The figure shows the increase in complexity from peri-urban low-density settlements to more densely populated informal neighbourhoods in large cities. The number of puzzle pieces represents complexity, while the shading highlights the role U-CLTS can play in achieving inclusive, city-wide sanitation.

Understanding the characteristics of the area is critical when deciding on an approach (strategies and methodology). In low-density peri-urban areas and smaller rural towns, where space exists and people are owner-occupiers, U-CLTS can play a more prominent role and an approach closer to the conventional rural CLTS methodology could be used. However, there needs to be consideration of whether the local government has aspirations for the area to become a higher-status settlement and to develop improved services.

In denser and more challenging urban environments, more adaptations will be needed compared with the rural approach. Also, any community-led intervention will need to be integrated with government and other stakeholders' plans into a larger, more complex programme.

In the most challenging areas, the tools and tactics outlined in this guide can be used to help increase participation and to help make existing approaches, systems, and frameworks more effective in delivering inclusive sanitation services.

LOW DENSITY / PERI-URBAN

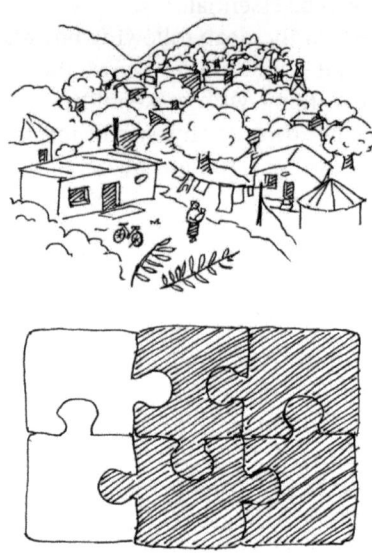

Urban typology	Low density/peri-urban
Characteristics	• Could be part of a small/medium town, large village or the outskirts of a medium to large city. • Urban and rural characteristics. • Space for household toilet construction.
Sanitation challenges	• Substantial proportion of OD. • Fixed-point OD/unimproved toilets. • Indiscriminate dumping when latrines emptied.
Associated case study	• Case Study 1: Choma, Zambia; • Case Study 3: Fort Dauphin Madagascar; • Case Study 4: Gulariya, Nepal; • Case Study 6: Himbirti, Eritrea; • Case Study 7: Iringa, Tanzania; • Case Study 10: Logo, Nigeria; • Case Study 13: New Delhi; • Case Study 14: Ribaué and Rapale, Mozambique; • Case Study 15: Small towns in Southern and Northern Nigeria.

Figure 1.3 Characteristics of different urban typologies and the associated U-CLTS case study
Source: CLTS Knowledge Hub. Illustration by Jamie Eke.

INTRODUCTION 9

SMALL / MEDIUM SIZED TOWNS

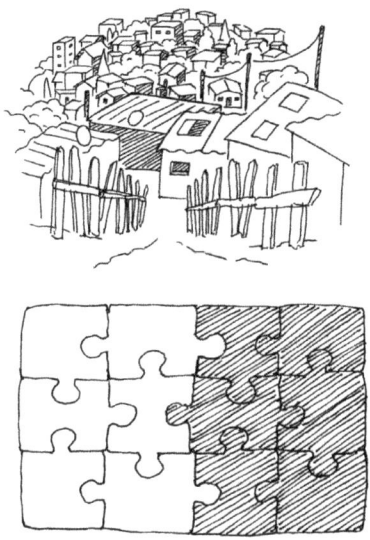

Urban typology	Small and medium sized towns/cities
Characteristics	• Less densely populated than larger cities – though population density in the centre is likely to be high. • May have networked water services.
Sanitation challenges	• Less OD. • Fixed-point OD. • Poorly built, maintained and cleaned compound, public and/or communal latrines. • Basic or unimproved household latrines. • Either lack safe FSM services or unserved by FSM services.
Associated case study	• Case Study 1: Choma, Zambia; • Case Study 2: Eight towns in Ethiopia; • Case Study 3: Fort Dauphin, Madagascar; • Case Study 4: Gulariya, Nepal; • Case Study 5: Hawassa, Ethiopia; • Case Study 6: Himbirti, Eritrea; • Case Study 9: Kabwe, Zambia; • Case Study 10: Logo, Nigeria; • Case Study 14: Ribaué and Rapale, Mozambique; • Case Study 15: Small towns in Southern and Northern Nigeria.

Figure 1.3 (continues)

FORMALISED NEIGHBOURHOOD

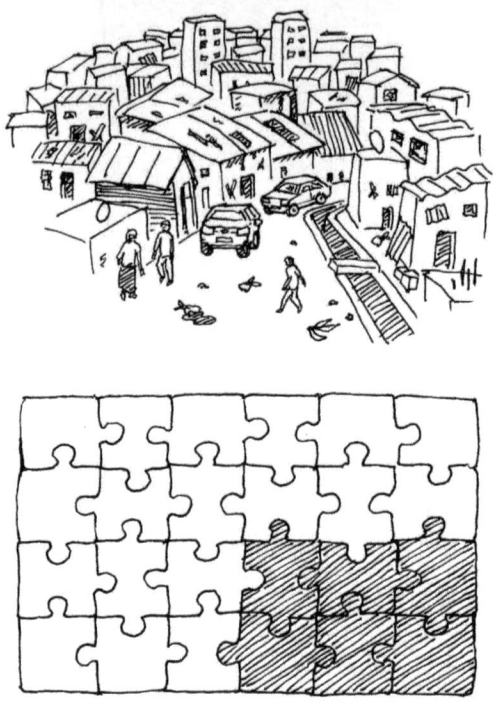

Urban typology	Formalized neighbourhoods of large cities
Characteristics	• Densely populated. • Likely to have basic networked services, at least water. • Security of tenure likely, may be owner occupied or rented out.
Sanitation challenges	• Little to no OD – perhaps some hotspots. Out of necessity rather than choice. • Fixed-point OD. • Poorly built, maintained and cleaned compound, public and/or communal latrines. • Basic or unimproved household latrines. • May have access to FSM services, if they exist.
Associated case study	• Case Study 8: IUWASH, Indonesia.

Figure 1.3 (continues)

INFORMAL NEIGHBOURHOOD

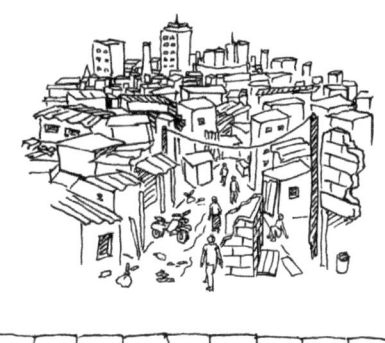

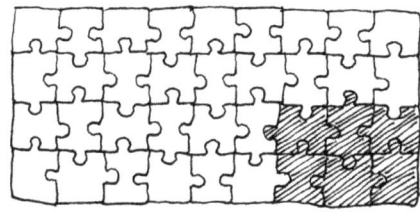

Urban typology	Informal neighbourhoods of large cities
Characteristics	• Densely populated. • Insecure land tenure likely. • Piped water, sewerage unlikely. • Many tenants in informal renting arrangements. • May not be recognized by government.
Sanitation challenges	• Little to no OD – perhaps some hotspots. Out of necessity rather than choice. • Fixed-point OD. • Flying toilets. • Poorly built, maintained and cleaned household, compound, public and/or communal latrines. • Hanging toilets. • Unserved by safe FSM services: i.e. full/overflowing pit latrines and septic tanks, households emptying tanks in the open, service providers indiscriminately dumping sludge.
Associated case study	• Case Study 8: IUWASH, Indonesia; • Case Study 11: Mathare 10, Nairobi, Kenya; • Case Study 12: Nakuru, Kenya;

Figure 1.3 (continued)

Challenges for U-CLTS

There are numerous persistent challenges to the development of affordable and inclusive urban sanitation infrastructure and services. These have been written about in detail and include: population density; lack of tenure security; poor definition of institutional roles and a lack of coordination; weak capacity; unused infrastructure; lack of investment; little to no regulation or enforcement; and limited human resource capacity (see Hawkins et al., 2013; Blackett et al., 2014). These make urban sanitation planning complex, time-consuming, and highly political, as mentioned earlier in the chapter. U-CLTS is not being proposed as a solution to all challenges but as an important part of the puzzle.

U-CLTS, and greater community participation in general, has the potential to respond to common challenges found in more conventional infrastructure-heavy sanitation programmes. U-CLTS tools have the potential to improve engagement and sustainability, for example by increasing ownership, reducing costs through community construction, and ensuring that toilets are used, maintained, and upgraded over time. New hurdles are likely to become more apparent when using a participatory, community-based approach. These include the following:

- *Changing mindsets about U-CLTS.* Sanitation in urban areas is often seen as an engineering problem by public health bodies, civil engineers, and planners. Communities can be seen as the unit of service delivery or as recipients of services. Urban sanitation stakeholders will need evidence to convince them that U-CLTS is useful and different from rural CLTS practice and has been adequately adapted to the needs and circumstances of urban areas.
- *Institutional arrangements.* The complexity of the urban setting and the sanitation chain means that a detailed understanding of the context is needed. This includes understanding the range of institutions and stakeholders and the overlaps and gaps in roles and responsibilities, as well as relevant local regulations, norms, and environmental sanitation plans.
- *Time and cost.* It will be much more expensive to resolve the challenges and bottlenecks for obtaining a shit-free environment than in rural areas. An analysis of the costs of U-CLTS relative to other urban interventions has yet to be done. So far, there has been limited experience or analysis, and, as a result, this is not tackled thoroughly in this guide.
- *Lack of documented evidence.* To date, approaches to and experiences with U-CLTS have been ad hoc rather than systematic. The range of participatory tools and methods described are based on current experience and can help provide useful ideas, recommendations, and practical steps.
- *Turning demand into access.* It is not always possible for community demand creation to result in rapid action by local governments and service providers, no matter how motivated the local government may be. For example, it may take time to clarify which institution is responsible

for which part of the sanitation chain, or to update regulations and access additional capacity and budgets. Communities and other facilitators will need to engage with and lobby a range of stakeholders and work with them over time to solve the real challenges and work towards appropriate solutions.
- *Practicalities of U-CLTS process*. There are a number of challenges associated with the practical implementation of the U-CLTS process (see Table 1.3). The list below is not exhaustive and it is important to carefully consider context-specific challenges.

Table 1.3 Some practical challenges of U-CLTS implementation

Challenge	Details
Community attendance at triggering	Busy lifestyles, based on the cash economy of urban dwellers, can mean low attendance at triggering. Meetings in the evening and at weekends will be more effective than during Monday–Friday business hours – although many people are still working then.
Working with local leaders	It is important to work with leaders who have influence in communities. Factors to consider include: • the fact that there may be a multitude of leaders (traditional, social, political, religious) who wield different influencing powers and often have competing interests within a community; • their limited presence in, interest in, or influence over communities; • the complexity of communities where users of improved sanitation are often not the investors (i.e. landlords providing – or not providing – a toilet, service providers improving their level of FSM services, government investing in public toilets, etc.).
Lack of social capital	Triggering and follow-up alone cannot overcome an existing lack of community capital. Social capital is likely to have an important role in levels of participation at community-wide triggering activities and action planning.
Working in informal areas	Households may not have land tenure in informal areas, and, as a result, the area may not be recognized by government; in such cases, the provision of services is not supported or encouraged. However, semi-legal housing or communities seeking legal status are common.
Integration with urban sanitation programmes	The provision of safe sanitation infrastructure and services in urban areas is a complex matter and many projects may be already happening – especially in larger cities. Communities will need to take an opportunistic approach and make a significant effort to integrate U-CLTS approaches into such interventions and wider sanitation improvement programmes.
Affordability is challenging	Safer toilet designs that are suitable for dense urban settings are often more expensive and households alone are unlikely to be able to bear the full costs without support. Emptying services, where available, also add costs to household budgets. Smaller pits can reduce the latrine costs, but they increase the frequency of emptying. More people requiring emptying may increase competition and economies of scale and hence reduce prices – but this cannot necessarily be assumed.

Table 1.4 Challenges and opportunities for using a U-CLTS approach

Challenging settings	Favourable settings	Ideal settings
• Weak or highly uninterested government institutions and/or sanitation stakeholders with other major priorities. • Short-term residents/tenants. • Gangs that control services in slums. • Lack of space to build household toilets or necessary FSM infrastructure. • Multi-storey dwellings. • Little to no understanding among programme/project/intervention implementers about potential solutions.	• Gaps in sanitation coverage. • Willingness and capacity of leaders/institutions/service providers. • Some community structures in place. • Visible missing links across the sanitation/faecal sludge chain. • Critical mass of owner-occupied permanent residences, with toilets or space to build them. • Existing sanitation infrastructure which is not fully used, operated, or well maintained. • Affordable, safe, and clean public toilets available nearby.	• Existing service providers. • Supply chains. • Government willing to support U-CLTS. • Failure of past supply-led approaches. • Sanitation a priority for the community. • Strategy or plan for U-CLTS. • A range of potential solutions exist to tackle the sanitation challenges. • Appropriate funds are available.

In some situations, U-CLTS will be more challenging while in other situations it will be more feasible (see Table 1.4). Using U-CLTS in some neighbourhoods may be appropriate, but in other neighbourhoods other approaches will be more effective. However, there is no context in which some form of community engagement in improving sanitation is not possible or relevant.

Roles and responsibilities within U-CLTS

Communities or households alone are unlikely to have the capacity, skills, financial resources, authority, or land to implement all aspects of a community action plan. Reasons for this are presented below:

- Municipal standards of toilet construction may be well beyond the capacity of residents, tenants, or landlords, leading to failure to comply.
- There may be inadequate space for some or all households to construct household latrines.
- Latrines may be full but cannot be emptied for reasons such as lack of access or suitable equipment, no FSM services available, or the FSM services are unaffordable.
- Landlords may be unwilling to build latrines. Tenants may lack authority and resources to do so, and also lack the power to require the landlords to do so. Tenants may also not want landlords to build latrines for fear of increased rents.
- A lack of understanding of the needs, capacity, or purchasing power of communities may lead technology and service providers to offer inappropriate options.

- Service providers may have limited knowledge of different options, possibly because such options have not yet been used in the country.
- Houses could be in challenging environments where pits cannot be dug or pipes easily laid: for example, on stilts over water, on steep rocky hillsides, or in frequently flooded areas.

It is therefore important to acknowledge that there are likely to be different roles and responsibilities within the U-CLTS process that extend well beyond the community.

More systematic attention to the sanitation chain is required – and to the service providers, the stakeholders, and broader urban development plans. Table 1.5 provides a simple outline of the generic roles and responsibilities, the realities will be much more complex.

Table 1.5 Roles and responsibilities of different sanitation stakeholders

Stakeholder role	Responsibility
Government, including national and municipal government, several different departments, utilities, etc.	• A system-wide approach that tackles several dimensions simultaneously, including policy, financing, institutions, and other key functions of the WASH-enabling environment. • Enforced laws and regulations. • Appropriate options for collection, treatment, disposal, or reuse of excreta. • Regulatory framework. • Government budget allocation/budget utilization. • Tracking of financial flows. • City investment plans. • Capacity of key institutions and service providers. • High-level political commitment. • National policy.
Private sector	• Provision of sanitation services and products. • Affordable financial services. • Business development support. • Research and development support.
International, national, and local NGOs	• Building capacity and skills of local actors and communities to deliver U-CLTS, and facilitating the U-CLTS process. • Liaison between different stakeholder groups. • Behaviour change campaigns. • Monitoring systems. • Inclusion of vulnerable and marginalized households.
Community-based organizations or Natural Leaders	• Facilitation of local action. • Monitoring of progress. • Maintaining enthusiasm. • Lobbying government and service providers and holding them to account. • Civil society voice.
Community	• Taking action within their capacity, e.g. building latrines where possible, cleaning up existing facilities, articulating their needs, lobbying government and service providers, and holding them to account. • Willingness to pay.

How to use this guide

The objective of this guide is to propose a framework, tools, and tactics geared to understanding, exploring, and implementing U-CLTS. It also aims to improve readers' knowledge of the added value of integrating U-CLTS into existing urban sanitation approaches, systems, and frameworks. It covers a range of urban settings, drawing on examples of effective and promising practices that can be adopted and adapted in different contexts.

The guide brings together a variety of individual tools that support the process of U-CLTS. The tools themselves are synthesized from real-world experience and derived from a review of literature and case studies. Those included in the guide are drawn from U-CLTS programmes or are examples of tools and tactics that adhere to overarching principles (see Chapter 1 section 'The principles of U-CLTS').

These ideas are intended to serve as inspiration for those wanting to design tools and processes that adhere to similar principles. U-CLTS is fairly new and there is growing, but relatively limited, experience so far. We do not have proven answers for every scenario, and we would like to see lessons learned built on field experience, implementation, reflection, and revision.

The guide is divided into two parts. Part 1 provides an introduction and overview of U-CLTS. It is intended to improve readers' knowledge of the added value of U-CLTS to existing urban sanitation approaches. It provides suggestions on how to design a U-CLTS programme or intervention as well as a number of tools for users, implementers, and regulators of urban sanitation. The focus in this section is on **what is needed**, **what to do**, and **why**, as well as **how to do it**. It includes a set of guiding principles, a collection of tools and tactics, and helpful resources. These tools and tactics provide guidance on the sequence of steps in U-CLTS:

- *Stage 1: Assessment and preparation (pre-triggering)*. Researching the local government responsibilities for sanitation and plans for housing, water and sanitation; building rapport with relevant stakeholders; situation analysis; stakeholder analysis; selecting communities; engaging partners; capacity building; preparing to enter communities.
- *Stage 2: U-CLTS triggering and institutional advocacy*. Participatory sanitation profile analysis; community triggering/ignition moment; community-led action planning; advocating institutions.
- *Stage 3: Integrating U-CLTS across the sanitation chain*. Safe capture and containment – facilitating supply; safe emptying and transportation; treatment and potential reuse; dealing with drainage and associated waste streams.
- *Stage 4: Maintaining momentum*. Scaling up; follow-up and monitoring; verification, certification and celebration.

Tools and tactics are presented throughout the document in order to provide ideas on how to implement U-CLTS in practice. The selection of tools will

Table 1.6 Tools and tactics listed under each stage

Stage 1: Assessment and preparation (pre-triggering)	Stage 3: Integrating U-CLTS across the sanitation chain
• Baseline surveys • Household enumeration surveys • Venn diagram mapping • Political economy analysis • Social network mapping	• Participatory technology development • Participatory tools for socially inclusive design • Participatory analysis of market systems for sanitation • Supply chain analysis • Solid waste calculations

Stage 2: U-CLTS triggering and institutional advocacy	Stage 4: Maintaining momentum
• Sanitation street theatre • Triggering homogeneous groups • Mob triggering • Plot/compound triggering • Sanitation mapping • Shit calculation • Household medical expenses calculations • Transect walk • Shit and water • Faecal oral contamination routes • Participatory video/photography • Analysing water contamination • Scenario planning • Ranking and prioritization tool • Sanitation Master Plans/City Sanitation Plans • Faecal waste/shit flow diagram • Sharing community triggering with key stakeholders • Exposure visits • Sharing the numbers • Landlord forums	• Sanitation ambassadors • Community exchange visits • Use of traditional and social media • Women's groups • Visual monitoring • Institutional performance scoring • Community scorecards • Inter-community monitoring • Mobile phone monitoring • Celebrating progress • Advertising hoardings

be dictated by the reader's context and purpose. Although the tools have been grouped into stages, there are obvious links between them.

Part 2 provides a description of 15 case studies that describe the use of the tools and tactics in a range of locations. The focus in this section is on **how others have done it**. The cases are to provide inspiration and ideas rather than to be copied. We expect this section to be added to with time as we gain more experience.

The guide deliberately avoids taking a blueprint or top-down approach, but rather takes the perspective of communities. By taking these tools and examples, and relating them systematically to various aspects of U-CLTS implementation, it should fulfil the urgent need expressed by policymakers and professional staff for advice on U-CLTS in the context of the SDGs. It has been deliberately designed to be as interactive as possible. Please use the 'notes' pages following each chapter to write down your ideas.

It is hoped that others will be encouraged to try these approaches, to learn and document their experiences, and to help improve and refine guidance in

> **Box 1.2 Guide to boxes and tables**
>
> **Dos and don'ts:** These tables are found at the end of each chapter. They are there to highlight both what is needed and what should be avoided.
>
> **Examples:** Examples have been drawn predominantly from U-CLTS programmes; however, examples from other programmes that are highly compatible with the tools and tactics listed and the defining principles have also been used (see Chapter 1 section 'The principles of U-CLTS'). Many of these refer to the case studies featured in Part 2. These boxes are dark grey.
>
> **Tips:** Tip boxes are found throughout the text and cover topics such as vulnerability, emerging questions, and key considerations. These boxes are light grey.
>
> **Blank pages:** The guide has been designed to be interactive. Blank pages are provided at the end of each chapter for readers to add their thoughts, ideas, and questions.

the future through documentation, critical reflection, and sharing. Readers should be able to dip in and out, and to selectively look up tools, case studies, and reference materials to assist with specific tasks.

This guide is a first attempt at providing global guidance on how U-CLTS can be adapted and used in urban settings. It is not an authoritative collection or a step-by-step instructional manual; rather, it is intended to be a working document and new tools and experiences can be added when they come to light.

Dos and don'ts

Table 1.7 General dos and don'ts for U-CLTS

Dos	*Don'ts*
1. Consider the U-CLTS principles and adapt approaches, tools, and tactics found throughout this guide to the local urban context.	1. Copy and paste the rural CLTS approach.
	2. Focus solely on OD and household latrines.
2. Find out what is needed and affordable aspirations (FSM, sewer connections, household, shared, or communal toilets) and be clear what possible options exist.	3. Assume the government is doing nothing to provide services, or has no plans.
	4. Assume urban people living in poverty cannot find some way to contribute to the programme or towards improving their sanitation situation.
3. Consider the urban typology and the role U-CLTS can play in relation to the challenges faced. A programme in a small rural town will be very different from an intervention in a poor and unserved part of a megacity such as Dhaka or Lagos.	5. Think that households do not have a latrine or that households are necessarily unable to build a latrine.
	6. Work in isolation from other development partners and government agencies and sanitation programmes.
4. Recognize that community settlement patterns, tenure, or density are critical and that they will change over the next two to 10 years.	7. Assume that others in the sector are conversant and confident about U-CLTS and that they understand U-CLTS terminology.

Table 1.7 General dos and don'ts for U-CLTS (*continued*)

Dos	Don'ts
5. Establish links, partner, and collaborate with those already working on urban sanitation (including local government, utilities, development partners, masons, sanitation marketing, loan-giving bodies, service providers, etc.).	
6. Develop a strategy/framework to guide actions on U-CLTS and against which actions and outcomes can be monitored.	
7. Develop activity checklist tools for assessment and preparation, triggering, actions across the sanitation chain, and maintaining momentum.	
8. Provide substantial, repeated capacity building on U-CLTS for urban sanitation stakeholders. Once is not enough.	
9. Advocate with government, development partners and other organizations to ensure that the potential benefits of U-CLTS are recognized in WASH policies, strategies, guidelines, national training guidance, and programmes.	
10. Document and share your experience: what you did and the learning from this.	
11. Contribute U-CLTS approaches to support other sanitation initiatives – they often lack knowledge of good participatory approaches.	

Notes for users

PART 1
The guide

CHAPTER 2
Stage 1: Assessment and preparation (pre-triggering)

Abstract

Urban communities can rarely achieve total safely managed sanitation without collaboration with a wide range of stakeholders. Assessment and preparation is the stage at which a U-CLTS team or facilitators analyse the broader context within which the urban community lives and then develops a sanitation profile, by collecting relevant information to support the U-CLTS process, finding out what else is happening and what is needed, and reflecting on how a U-CLTS approach can be applied. Gaining a deeper and comprehensive understanding of the context – i.e. the community, sanitation service issues, stakeholders, ongoing interventions, etc. – will inform the design of effective U-CLTS processes and how they can be integrated into the wider urban environment. This chapter describes the information that needs to be collected and how to go about collecting this. It includes ideas for both situational and stakeholder analyses, both of which are needed to design subsequent phases of the U-CLTS process.

Keywords: situational analysis, stakeholder analysis, collaboration, U-CLTS, sanitation profile, safely managed sanitation

Key messages

- Assessment and preparation is the stage at which a U-CLTS team or facilitators collect relevant information to support the U-CLTS process, find out what else is happening and what is needed, and reflect on how U-CLTS approaches can be applied.
- The range and roles of different stakeholders must be understood early on in the process so that they can be integrated into the assessment and preparation, triggering, and actions needed across the sanitation service chain.
- Actions by the community alone cannot deliver all aspects of safely managed sanitation in urban areas. A good understanding of the complexities of relevant institutions, the institutional overlaps and gaps, and their current and future plans, challenges, and approaches is needed. U-CLTS is there to help them, and their support and commitment is important. This requires working in partnership with the relevant local

institutional leaders mandated to ensure good urban sanitation: for example, municipal departments, local government agencies, water and sewerage utilities, and other local service providers.
- Once institutional stakeholders are interested and supportive, capacity building and preparation are required. This stage includes selecting communities; identifying possible feasible sanitation options; training facilitators in the U-CLTS process; planning the U-CLTS strategy; baseline data collection; etc.
- This stage also requires preparation of the community and local leadership for implementation of the U-CLTS triggering and the subsequent processes.

Purpose of assessment and preparation

The overall objective of this phase is to jointly analyse the broader context within which the urban community lives and to develop a sanitation profile: i.e. a list of existing initiatives, practices, constraints/challenges, opportunities, and national and local plans and budgets, and an assessment of how these contribute to the existing urban sanitation situation. This information should assist in the selection of communities, form the basis for building positive relationships with and between stakeholders, and inform the strategy for triggering actions across the sanitation chain and maintaining momentum. In some cases, relevant reports may already exist and should not be repeated.

The purpose of this stage is to gain a deeper and more comprehensive understanding of the context – the community, sanitation service issues, stakeholders, ongoing interventions, etc. – to inform the design of effective U-CLTS processes and how they are integrated into the wider urban environment.

A U-CLTS approach views the community as the driver of action towards achieving total sanitation. However, communities can rarely achieve total safely managed sanitation without collaboration with a wider range of agencies, duty bearers, and the private sector. Therefore, alongside the triggering of communities to take action, an urban approach will also need engaged institutions to respond to community needs and demands.

More extensive preparation is therefore needed to understand both the broader urban community and the institutional context and thus ensure that all subsequent stages are appropriate and involve the right people. A thorough assessment of the context and preparation will improve the chances of success in the triggering and other subsequent phases.

This phase involves:

- *Situation analysis.* To better understand the nature and dynamics of the selected area in terms of population, tenancy, migration, housing, organization, etc.; to determine the nature, magnitude, and multiple causes of sanitation problems; and to evaluate what changes are needed and assess the feasible options along the sanitation chain.
- *Stakeholder analysis and identifying key partners.* To map institutional stakeholders and their roles and responsibilities in relation to implementing,

maintaining, and managing sanitation services, and to start building links with them.
- *Selection of communities and partner capacity building.* To apply the above information to engage appropriate key local partners in the process; select specific communities for intervention; and make appropriate preparations for triggering – for example, engaging local leadership, selecting suitable days and times for meetings.
- *Preparing to enter the community.* To engage local leadership and make arrangements for the triggering phase to begin.

Assessing vulnerability

> **Tip 2.1 – Consider vulnerability**
>
> Vulnerabilities can be accentuated in urban areas. In rural areas communities may have similar work, ideas, values, interests, and norms of behaviour. In urban areas there can be a variety of jobs, lifestyles, values, and aspirations.
>
> Vulnerability could relate to any of the following inequalities:
>
> - Individual-related inequalities are based on gender, age and disability, marital and family status, sexual orientation and gender identity, health status, ownership of property, and people's economic and social situation.
> - Group-related inequalities are based on race, colour, ethnicity, language, religion, political persuasion, national or social origin, caste, or migratory status.
> - Geographic inequalities are based on the place of residence: e.g. between formal and informal settlements.
>
> *Source*: Committee on Economic, Social and Cultural Rights (CESCR), General Comment No. 20 on non-discrimination, UN Doc. E/C.12/GC/20, 2009.
>
> People who are in vulnerable and/or marginalized situations may:
>
> - be less visible;
> - have less of a voice and less confidence to speak in public;
> - be less likely or able to demand their rights;
> - not be listened to;
> - have less time available for community activities;
> - be under-represented in policy and decision-making, and face barriers accessing public institutions due to language, culture, or racism;
> - not be able to read or write easily;
> - live on the edge of communities with less access to services;
> - face stigma or prejudice;
> - have less access to finances and resources, and may be unable to provide cash or labour contributions;
> - have different beliefs, cultures or practices to the majority;
> - have different needs, including relating to WASH; and/or
> - have less access to information (such as information on services, tariff structures, their rights and entitlements as per national policy and international laws, and mechanisms to make complaints and claim their rights).
>
> *Source*: House et al., 2014.

Box 2.1 Implications of vulnerability for U-CLTS

There are a number of factors that affect an individual's or a group's ability to participate in U-CLTS processes or construct, access, use, or maintain a latrine. In particular, **physical ability**, **access to income and assets**, and **support from family members** have a significant impact on whether a person will need support from within or outside the community. Using the 'Clusters of disadvantage' (Figure 2.1) can help show how these challenges overlap and are interrelated. For example, if you are a person with disabilities or an older person heading a household, but have a business or a lot of savings, you are still likely to be able to construct a latrine that you can access and use. People who fall into more than one group are likely to be most disadvantaged (e.g. a widowed older woman with limited or no savings and no regular income looking after grandchildren alone and living in a flood-affected area).

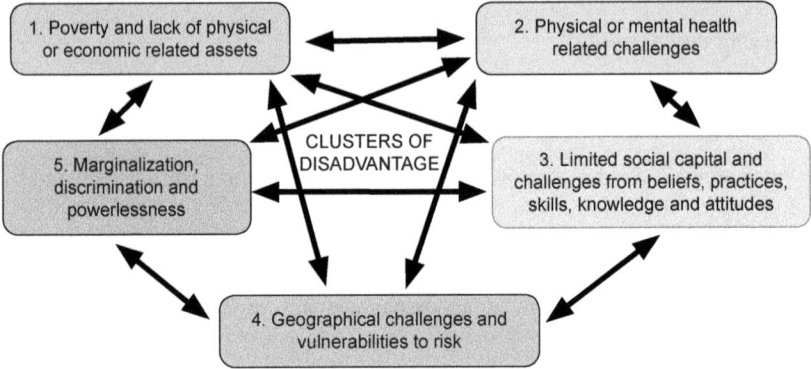

Figure 2.1 Clusters of disadvantage
Note: a) The arrows indicate the interconnectedness of each factor to the other factors; b) An individual or group affected by more than one factor is likely to be more advantaged than an individual or group affected by just one; c) This figure has been adapted from Chambers' (1983) analysis of the deprivation trap related to rural communities.
Source: House et al., 2017.

The implications of such inequalities for sanitation include safety, convenience, ease of use, self-esteem, health, dignity, and improved environment. For instance, there may be a number of barriers to vulnerable people's engagement in U-CLTS:

- exclusion from pre-triggering or triggering U-CLTS processes;
- inability to pay for construction or FSM services or use assets to build toilets;
- experience of coercive pressure or humiliation to comply with community demands for ODF;
- inability to pay to use public toilets (e.g. among transient or homeless populations);
- barriers to the access and use of latrines for individuals within households (e.g. disabled or elderly people);
- exclusion from the use of community or public facilities (e.g. among transgender women); and/or
- lack of attention to feelings of safety around toilet use.

Designing U-CLTS programmes that ensure full social inclusion in terms of people's ability to construct, access, and maintain sanitation and handwashing facilities requires attention to vulnerability from the start and throughout the process, i.e. in stakeholder analysis, enforcing regulations, monitoring, etc.

Strengthening the capacity of U-CLTS facilitators and community WASH management systems and investing in community groups (such as women's groups or organizations representing people with disabilities) can ensure more community solidarity and improved U-CLTS-related processes. A focus on small, immediate, and doable actions together with access to financial and other support can help ensure that vulnerable people can construct, access, and maintain toilets and handwashing facilities, and sustain behaviours.

Example 2.1 – Considering vulnerability and planning for safety

Involving adolescent girls in assessing safety: Adolescent girls participated in Plan Peru's Safer Cities workshops to identify violence-related problems and how young people feel about insecurities in their communities. This involved the girls undertaking a range of exercises including social cartography (mapping) and the development of girls' opportunity stars and girls' safety walks. The workshops led to girls identifying priority issues that they would like to be addressed and their recommendations.

Source: Plan International et al., 2013.

Integrating women's safety concerns into urban services, India: Jagori, Women in Cities International, ActionAid India, and partners worked with women, men, and adolescent/teenage girls and boys to investigate the security concerns of each group, and supported community members to engage with the authorities to look for solutions. The process of investigating safety issues included a mapping of services and identification of problem areas, focus group discussions, a safety audit walk, and in-depth interviews with women. This initial learning was followed by a capacity-building programme to develop a core team of community members (women and female and male youth) who were then able to mobilize the community and local government. The capacity-building efforts aimed to build self-esteem, improve people's ability to challenge power relations, and promote leadership and learning from other community-led interventions. The male and female youth also prepared a radio programme based on interviews with local people. This was used to promote discussions with groups of community members in the vicinity to increase understanding and encourage changes in behaviours.

Source: Women in Cities International et al., 2011.

Situation analysis

The first part of the situation analysis will provide the information necessary to determine and confirm the sanitation needs of the community and to assess if and how U-CLTS tools can assist in addressing them. It will also help understand the ongoing or planned sanitation initiatives that may be happening and how U-CLTS can contribute towards these.

It is also essential to assess what the feasible sanitation chain options are – this does not mean that communities need to be told about them, but they must realistically exist and be affordable. Do people have the authority to build latrines on their plots? Are they the owners of the land and houses or are they tenants? Are they living there legally? Is there space to build latrines – or rebuild them? If latrines exist, are they used? And if not, why not? Are there any accessible public or community toilets? Are they used by men, women, children, disabled people, etc.? Are pit latrines emptied? If so, how and by whom? Where does the sludge go? If there a treatment facility? How far away is it?

As part of this phase, it is necessary to be clear about government and development partners' plans for the area. For example, is the area due for upgrading, clearance, or redevelopment? What is the water supply situation, and are there plans to improve it? Where is the nearest sewer, if there are any? Are there available FSM services for emptying, transport, and treatment?

If the community is suitable and it has been agreed to use U-CLTS, then the second stage will involve developing appropriate triggering and follow-up strategies. A situation analysis should cover elements important for programme design and methodologies for implementation. It is important to gain a sound understanding of the following aspects:

- basic demographics of the area, including socioeconomic status, disease, culture, disability, vulnerability/poverty, marginalized groups, etc.;
- land ownership, plot layout, and tenancy arrangements;
- settlement patterns and topography;
- information on the availability, access, and use of different forms of sanitation or sanitation-related services;
- incomes, rents, and costs of accessing sanitation (both shared and household) and related services;
- existing service providers for FSM, solid and liquid waste management, cleaning services, etc.;
- access to water, waste, and storm water drainage and solid waste management;
- other infrastructure such as roads, which are particularly relevant for FSM;
- attitudes to WASH to help inform any behaviour change communications campaigns;
- problems across the entire sanitation chain from containment to disposal – i.e. existing latrine coverage, usage, maintenance, and other practices relating to hygiene such as handwashing, school sanitation, etc.;
- how the area/community fits into the larger urban system; and
- strategic or other relevant investment plans by government and/or its partners.

Situation analysis should draw on existing data from existing reports, local authorities, surveys, and other documents. These could include:

- previous government or development partner reports, or NGO sanitation project reports, including backgrounds, baselines, and evaluations;
- local/municipal government databases or data sources for relevant themes; and
- national population and local health census data.

Desk-based analysis could be complemented or verified by key informant interviews: for example, with municipal departments (both leadership and staff), representatives of service providers (public and private), any development partner projects, NGOs, community-based organizations (CBOs), and other local institutions and leaders.

STAGE 1: ASSESSMENT AND PREPARATION (PRE-TRIGGERING)   29

There are numerous ways in which information can be collected. The two examples presented below are baseline surveys and household numeration surveys (Tool 2.1 and 2.2, and Example 2.3 and 2.4). These can be used in conjunction with one another. The questions for both surveys should be designed based on the aspects listed above. Before beginning, plan how to capture information specific to vulnerable and potentially disadvantaged groups.

TOOL 2.1 – Baseline survey

What is it?	Baseline surveys are an important part of any monitoring and evaluation (M&E) process. A baseline study is done at the beginning of a project to establish the current status of a population before a programme is rolled out. It might be a knowledge, attitudes, and perceptions (KAP) survey relating to the issue of sanitation in a local community.
Why use it?	A baseline study is essential to ensure that implementers are later able to measure the impact the project has had on the target community.
	The information can also be used to help design subsequent phases of the programme.
How to use it	The survey could be done in an interview, paper questionnaire, or phone or online survey. The availability of funds and time will dictate the intensity and scope of the baseline study.
	Findings should be utilized in subsequent planning.
When would you use it?	Baseline surveys should be carried out at the very beginning of a programme to enable the design of later stages. Where a baseline study is conducted after the programme has already begun, it is difficult to gain an accurate picture of impact.
Related case studies	Case Study 3: Fort Dauphin, Madagascar.
	Case Study 4: Gulariya, Nepal.

Example 2.2 – Baseline data collection

In the planning stages, SEED Madagascar engaged the heads of an urban fokontany (neighbourhood) and government health volunteers to collect data in targeted communities on knowledge, attitudes, and practices with respect to WASH, demographics, popular pastimes, influential figures, and town planning.

This enabled them to identify priority sites and communities where they could work, appropriate triggers, the type of support households may need, how to make activities fun, and when people were more likely to be available, as well as potential role models they could engage.

Source: Case Study 3: Fort Dauphin, Madagascar; Azafady, 2015.

TOOL 2.2 – Participatory household enumeration survey

What is it?	A detailed household-level survey that gathers socio-economic and demographic data (including employment status, education, access to government grants, access to basic services, access to government, social, and community infrastructure, etc.). It can involve high levels of participation from community members. When a mobilized community collects its own data, the data obtained reflects far higher degrees of accuracy than any census or survey run by 'outsiders'.
Why use it?	The enumerations provide an updated settlement profile that can form the basis for any future plans. The data collection exercise serves as a means of mobilizing communities, equipping members with accurate information that can be used to advocate for development priorities. When enumerations are conducted in partnership with poor communities, they help in gaining accurate and more comprehensive data that can be used to design subsequent phases.
	Networks of poor urban residents can consciously adopt strategies of self-enumeration that become powerful negotiation tools in their dealings with governments. Communities are best positioned to develop community development plans: residents have the most up-to-date knowledge on how many households make up their settlement, how long they have lived there, and how they make a living.
How to use it	Enumerators create a qualitative and quantitative map of their settlement. Their work is twofold: 1) to survey each household; and 2) to number and measure every structure. A subsequent verification process within the community enables areas of disagreement to be identified and mediated by community members.
	On the day of the enumeration, an enumeration team is elected and trained. The community discusses and prioritizes the breadth and depth of the types of knowledge they want to capture: e.g. vulnerable groups, safety and security, health and wellness, etc. This data is collected at the household level to give a comprehensive profile of the settlement.
When would you use it?	Prior to or soon after any triggering event, to inform future upgrading or community action plans.
Further guidance	Yap, 2015, https://assets.publishing.service.gov.uk/media/57a089e540f0b649740002f8/Chinhoyi_Zimbabwe_POLICY_BRIEF.pdf
	Walnycki and Schermbruker, 2016, https://www.shareresearch.org/research/how-collective-action-strategies-urban-poor-can-improve-access-sanitation

> **Example 2.3 – Enumeration surveys**
>
> In Shackleton, Chinoyi, Zimbabwe, as part of the Sanitation and Hygiene Applied Research for Equity (SHARE) project, Slum Dwellers International and their affiliates carried out household enumeration surveys. Data collected included the cost of water and sanitation, willingness to pay for services, and land tenure arrangements, as well as information on how willing community members were to participate in upgrading and managing improved water and sanitation facilities.
>
> The mapping and profiling were the beginning of the process to develop inclusive and sustainable sanitation strategies.
>
> *Source*: Yap, 2015.

Stakeholder analysis and identifying key partners

Community actions will not deliver all aspects of sanitation needs in urban areas without the involvement of the institutions that are responsible for such services and possibly other external support. Therefore, the range and roles of other sanitation actors must be understood early on in the process so that relationships and partnerships can be developed and they can be integrated into all stages.

A stakeholder analysis will help U-CLTS facilitators identify different actors and institutions and their roles and responsibilities across the sanitation service chain. The purpose is to understand who the formal and informal influential actors are, where they are located, and how they are influential.

Stakeholders include individuals, community leaders, groups, and other organizations that could benefit from U-CLTS, find it useful, or influence the outcome. Examples of stakeholders in urban sanitation include a range of people and institutions:

- *Responsible agencies*. These could include national ministries, regulatory agencies, various municipalities/local government departments, politicians, health and community development offices, ward and neighbourhood administrators, mandated public service providers, and public water and sewerage utilities and regulators. These may exist, but it is more likely that responsibilities will need further clarification for the various steps along the sanitation chain. Please note, these may exist, but it is more likely that responsibilities will need further clarification for the various steps along the sanitation chain.
- *Development partners*. These may be involved in projects on urban water supply and sanitation, urban upgrading, and housing programmes. They could include development banks, bilateral development agencies, multilateral and UN agencies, and NGOs.
- *Academic and research bodies*. In some situations, research and piloting may be undertaken by national and international agencies.

- *The private sector*. This would include local, national, and international sanitation service providers (licensed/formal and unlicensed/informal), financial institutions (banks as well as microfinance institutions), and private water and sewerage companies.
- *Individuals and groups*. These could be: community leaders; vulnerable people; youth, women's, and disability groups; savings groups; informal-sector workers (including those offering FSM services); CBOs; landlords' and tenants' associations; religious leaders; and staff working in clinics and schools.

Stakeholder analysis can take the form of interviews, focus group discussions, and/or workshops to ensure that all stakeholders are identified and the roles, characteristics, and relationships between them are understood. The tools below can help generate insights into the importance and influence of each stakeholder. With this information, it becomes possible to develop a specific approach and strategy for the identified stakeholders. Institutional analysis is an important element of stakeholder analysis. It is necessary to understand the 'rules of the game' – the existing policies and processes relating to solid waste management, water service provision, waste water management, and FSM across the entire sanitation chain – that will influence stakeholder decisions or constraints. It is also important to be clear about all existing projects, plans, and strategies in the housing, water, and sanitation sectors that could impact the community and the surrounding communities.

The stakeholder analysis should naturally help identify key organizations to partner with initially in the U-CLTS triggering, and help guide the strategy for the longer-term delivery of improved sanitation services. Key partners are those whose buy-in and commitment are essential for engaging with the community around sanitation. They might include the municipal authority, the water utility, public and environmental health departments, the department of public works, a community development department, or locally active development projects, NGOs, CBOs, community champions, politicians, etc. Stakeholder analysis can also identify those who might stand to lose out and who might hinder or block the process, requiring action to get them on side.

At this point it may not be relevant to engage all sanitation-related agencies, as those that are relevant will emerge from the community triggering and community-led action planning stages (see Chapter 3).

TOOL 2.3 – Venn diagram mapping

What is it?	A review of key stakeholders and their relationships to each other, including the power dynamics. Also known as a chapati diagram, it can be used to identify and analyse institutions and relationships using symbols or circles (objects) of varying sizes to represent individuals, groups, or organizations and their perceived importance in a community or a given group of people.

Why use it?	It helps to understand the institutional arrangements within and beyond the community that have a responsibility for sanitation. This kind of mapping helps to understand the power and relationships between actors and institutions that can support or block improvements in sanitation. Analysing different power relations can help identify factors that might be preventing achievement of a shit-free environment and show how marginalized and disempowered people are excluded from decision-making on sanitation as well as from targets for advocacy and policy work.
How to use it	The size of the symbols/objects or circles used can be adapted to indicate the perceived power or importance of different institutions or actors. The positioning – overlapping, touching, or separate – indicates their degree of interaction. Key question to guide the process include the following: • Who are the key institutions (i.e. agencies, groups, individuals) in the community? What is the mandate (roles and responsibilities) for each of them in urban sanitation? • What is their relationship with the community and with each other? • How are the different actors perceived (relevance, performance, strengths, and weaknesses in relation to their role in urban sanitation)? • What power do they have? How have they used their power and with what effects on whom (effects could be negative or positive)? • What actions are needed to ensure that such institutions use their power and exercise their mandate responsibly for the benefit of the community as it relates to urban sanitation?
When would you use it?	At the beginning and throughout the process.
Further guidance	SSWM, n.d., https://www.sswm.info/content/venn-diagrams

TOOL 2.4 – Political economy analysis

What is it?	Political economy analysis (PEA) has been described as 'concerned with the interaction of political and economic processes in a society: the distribution of power and wealth between different groups and individuals, and the processes that create, sustain and transform these relationships over time' (ODI, 2009).

Why use it?	It can help generate context-specific responses by helping to explain why a sanitation situation is the way it is, identifying the drivers and bottlenecks for progress, and searching for win–win situations.
	It supports strategic reflection on the question of how change happens at the sector level, and what can drive the changes needed to achieve universal access. It can also be used for strategic reflection and for overcoming blockages when they occur.
How to use it	PEA involves working with different stakeholders to map out institutions (both formal and informal) and their specified and actual roles, and to highlight incentives and power that support or derail improvements in sanitation.
	Important questions to ask during the process include: • Who decides? • Who benefits? • Can things change? • What are the commonalities between interests? • Can groups be mobilized around them, and, if so, which groups?
	They are most effective when they focus on a particular topic rather than on sanitation in general, such as informal pit emptiers or managing communal latrines. Consequently, it may be appropriate to undertake a number of different PEAs on specific topics.
	By the end of the process there should be stakeholder agreement on important actions that are needed.
	A PEA can be a standalone assessment or performed in conjunction with other sector assessments tools such as WASH bottleneck analysis (WASH BAT) or the CLTS rapid assessment protocol (CRAP) tool.
When would you use it?	It can be used when designing and developing practical win–win scenarios, reviewing sectoral programmes, or influencing plans.
Further guidance	Coursera, n.d., https://www.coursera.org/learn/sanitation/lecture/HyysG/5-6-tools-for-institutional-and-political-economy-analysis-for-sanitation
	Kooy and Harris, 2012, https://www.odi.org/sites/odi.org.uk/files/odi-assets/publications-opinion-files/7797.pdf
	WASH BAT, 2016, http://www.washbat.org/

STAGE 1: ASSESSMENT AND PREPARATION (PRE-TRIGGERING)

> **Box 2.2 Political economy analysis for faecal sludge management**
>
> Prognosis for Change (PFC) assessments (PEA assessments that are sensitively addressed in order for the analysis to be shared and discussed among relevant stakeholders) have been developed to assess FSM service delivery. PFC assessments were conducted as part of a wider diagnostic for service delivery in five cities: Balikpapan in Indonesia, Dhaka in Bangladesh, Hawassa in Ethiopia, Lima in Peru, and Santa Cruz in Bolivia.
>
> The PFCs looked at how key formal and informal institutions function, what incentives institutions provide for different stakeholders, and the power of stakeholders in causing or preventing something from happening. PFCs include:
> - institutional mapping of FSM responsibilities;
> - stakeholder analysis and mapping; and
> - process mapping.
>
> They have been used to help explain why the current FSM situation is working (or not working) in the way it is, and to identify potential obstacles to progress. PFCs involve the collection of primarily qualitative data through key informant interviews and focus group discussions as well as secondary data from key sector documents, reports, and studies.
>
> *Source:* Ross et al., 2016a, 2016b.

TOOL 2.5 – Social network mapping

What is it? Social network mapping is the mapping and visualizing of the relationships and connections between people, groups, and organizations.

Why use it? To highlight the value of social networks, seeing how people connect and how these connections can be utilized to influence wide-scale action and behaviour change. It shows informal relationships – who knows who and who shares information and knowledge with whom.

Social contacts can play a critical role in achieving improved sanitation status. Social network mapping has been used to test whether an individual's social contacts are a significant predictor of individual latrine ownership. Individuals are more likely to own latrines if their social contacts own latrines. Social network mapping can be used to see how strong the social ties are between people in the community.

How to use it Key stages of the process typically include:
- identifying the network of people to be analysed;
- gathering names of the social contacts and any other relevant information;
- visually mapping the network (this can be done on paper or with a social mapping software tool); and
- designing and implementing actions to increase the improved sanitation uptake.

A social network map can be done alone, by researchers, with key stakeholders, with communities, or among the implementation team.

	The end product can help you identify key influencers in a community who can then help in the delivery of behaviour change communication messaging.
When would you use it?	Mapping during the assessment and preparation phase to identify who knows who and who knows what, and identifying key influencers.
Further guidance	Shakya et al., 2015, https://doi.org/10.1016/j.socscimed.2014.03.009
	Hanneman and Riddle, 2005, http://www.faculty.ucr.edu/~hanneman/nettext/
	Ebener, 2008, http://www1.paho.org/CDMEDIA/KMC-SNA/training-sna.htm

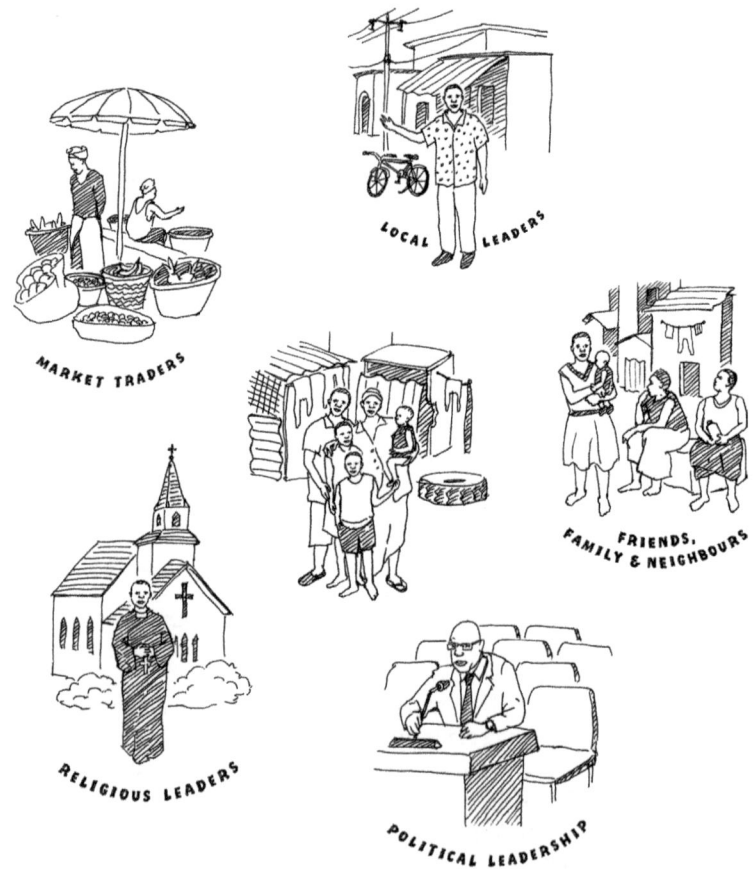

Figure 2.2 Potential key social influencers
Source: CLTS Knowledge Hub. Illustration by Jamie Eke.

> **Example 2.4 – Influencers from different U-CLTS programmes**
>
> *Religious leaders*
>
> In Nigeria, religious leaders have helped reinforce community decisions with reference to both Biblical and Quranic texts. By preaching sanitation and hygiene messages to their congregations in churches and mosques, religious leaders not only reinforce community decisions to adopt sanitation but also help to make the use of toilets and good hygiene practices a social norm. This is particularly true in an urban setting where congregations often attract worshippers from a number of different communities. But as institutions with buildings – churches and mosques – they can pose a challenge for implementation of U-CLTS if they do not provide toilets. In Cross River State, planning consent for new churches is refused if they are to be built without a latrine.
>
> *Motorcycle taxi riders*
>
> Motorcycle taxis, or *Okadas* as they are known in Nigeria, provide an essential public transport service, transporting people and goods between village and urban markets. Ugep Town is a hub from which many *Okadas* serve Yakurr Local Government Area (LGA). *Okada* riders are an important urban stakeholder group in the LGA-wide approach to CLTS. *Okadas* often carry people to and through communities; if they are not sensitized or 'triggered', they can unwittingly disrupt a shit-free environment by shitting in the bush. Some communities have set up public toilets to deal with this problem. Just as importantly, *Okada* riders transport hundreds of passengers every day and so can play a useful role in advocating for CLTS.
>
> *Source*: UNICEF Nigeria, 2014.

Key partner capacity building and selection of communities

Based on the findings of the situational and institutional analyses, potential partners are likely to emerge who will be able to play an active and/or supportive role in the U-CLTS process. Potential partners may be drawn from any of the stakeholder groups listed above in the section 'Stakeholder analysis and identifying key partners', such as relevant government departments, public or private service providers, NGOs, CBOs, political or local leaders, etc. They should be identified based on their potential contribution to the success of the U-CLTS process.

Once potential partners have been identified, it may require some additional advocacy or capacity building to ensure that they fully understand and support citizen-led efforts and the U-CLTS process. Those who understand and have buy-in to U-CLTS may be invited to join a taskforce or team to lead the U-CLTS process. They are fostered to become the institutional or individual champions for the process and will assist in ensuring that the environment is conducive.

> **Example 2.5 – Key partners**
>
> In Mathare 10, Kenya, the U-CLTS process was led by Plan International. They enlisted Community Cleaning Services, Nairobi City Council, and the Ministry of Public Health and Sanitation as key partners. Other champions emerged from the private sector, such as sanitation entrepreneurs, NGOs, human rights groups, and research institutions; their roles developed as the process continued.
>
> *Source*: Case Study 11: Mathare 10, Nairobi, Kenya.
>
> In Gulariya, Nepal, Practical Action worked through the municipal government to implement CLTS in a peri-urban context. They engaged municipal leadership through the project management committee and invested considerable effort in informing and engaging a wide range of stakeholders through training and workshops to ensure they fully understood the CLTS process. Pressure from national government to deliver on national sanitation goals complemented their local efforts and ODF was achieved in a population of 60,000, over 50 per cent of whom were practising OD in just six months.
>
> *Source*: Case Study 4: Gulariya, Nepal; Pasteur and Prabhakaran, 2015.

Building awareness, capacity and buy-in among relevant stakeholders is key to gaining their commitment and creating a more favourable enabling environment. Capacity building at this stage needs to provide a solid understanding that the U-CLTS objectives are not about toilet building but about a shit-free environment, the process, and the skills needed for facilitating, triggering, and community-led action planning.

U-CLTS interventions may adopt different approaches or strategies in different places, and there are no right or wrong ways to go about this. The key advice is to carefully consider the situation analysis, build strong local relationships, and take advice from the relevant stakeholders you have selected to engage with.

Preparing to enter the community

In urban settings, community dynamics are complex. While it may be easy to define and identify a community in the rural setting using geographical boundaries and shared resources, this may not be the case in urban settings.

Communities, or groups of people, in urban settings may be formed on the basis of common interests or jobs, or they may be migrants from a specific geographical area or 'communities of interest'. They may also be a heterogeneous group of people who have settled in one area. Depending on the history of the 'community', the bonds of trust and social capital may be high – or they may be low or non-existent. So, for U-CLTS, this means deciding what triggering strategy to take (see Chapter 3 section 'Triggering strategy'). People

STAGE 1: ASSESSMENT AND PREPARATION (PRE-TRIGGERING)

may have strong ties that are not based on geographic proximity: for example, people may not know their neighbours well but are closely linked through a church, fellow market traders, ethnicity, where they originated, or a savings group.

It is therefore important to start from the point of view that communities are not homogeneous. Facilitators need to understand how they are organized, and their power structures and power relations. This understanding will provide facilitators with an opportunity to learn how best to navigate through the structures and relate to the urban communities while ensuring equitable participation in decision-making in the U-CLTS process.

By understanding the community dynamics and power relations it will then be possible for the U-CLTS facilitation team to take decisions about what types of triggering will be needed: targeted, zoned neighbourhoods, or plot level (see Chapter 3 section 'Triggering strategy'). This will help identify appropriate entry points, build rapport, and develop communication processes in readiness for U-CLTS triggering.

Key tasks here will include exploratory visits to:

- identify different groups and structures and analyse the complex relationships that exist within the urban communities;
- understand power and power relations and other factors that could hinder or promote genuine participation during the U-CLTS process – and also identify vulnerable and potentially vulnerable groups;
- build relationships with a range of local leaders, groups, and other stakeholders that will facilitate smooth entry into the community for triggering; and
- develop strategies for reaching the maximum number of people and ensuring equal opportunities for participation during the triggering process.

These could be done through structured consultative meetings with key informants in the urban communities where U-CLTS will be undertaken.

Dos and don'ts for assessment and preparation (pre-triggering)

Table 2.1 Dos and don'ts: assessment and preparation

Dos	Don'ts
1. Review what information is already available – is there a need to update it or fill gaps? Plan and conduct preparatory visits for the purpose of learning.	1. Cut short the assessment – this is a vital stage of the process in U-CLTS.
2. Find out about all the other sanitation programmes happening in the areas and seek to work with them.	2. Neglect municipal and local government and local leadership – make sure they are ready to lead the way and be supportive of the process.

Table 2.1 Dos and don'ts: assessment and preparation (*continued*)

Dos	Don'ts
3. Conduct a situational and stakeholder analysis – consider roles, responsibilities, relationships, and power dimensions. 4. Identify different groups and segments within the community – focus on leadership, key influencers, and vulnerable groups. 5. Consider what options are feasible what changes can be community-led and what other stakeholders will have to support. Further information can be found at: http://www.communityledtotalsanitation.org/sites/communityledtotalsanitation.org/files/Supporting_the_least_able.pdf 6. Build networks, alliances, and connections with existing urban actors' programmes. 7. With the community leadership and representatives, identify those who might be disadvantaged or would be less likely to attend the triggering session – plan how to involve excluded groups in the process (i.e. people with disabilities, older people, male and female youth, minority groups, etc). 8. Involve women's and youth leaders as well as leaders from various community institutions in the pre-planning phase. 9. Develop a set of criteria for selecting and prioritizing communities. There must be a need and an expression of need from the community leadership. 10. Ensure that the timing of community profiling, analyses, and triggering are suitable for the community and its leadership. 11. Ensure that the necessary groundwork is done before entering the community. Conduct a WASH baseline assessment for planning and programming.	3. Ignore conflicts or power relations as they are likely to affect the U-CLTS process. 4. Think U-CLTS can be done in isolation. 5. Try to find out everything in the first instance – be focused and collect only relevant information.

Notes for users

CHAPTER 3
Stage 2: U-CLTS triggering and institutional advocacy

Abstract

Combining community and institutional action can lead to stronger accountability and the development of a shared realistic plan to achieve a shit-free environment. Yet how can communities, and other stakeholders, be mobilized to take action to address poor sanitation challenges facing their urban communities across the sanitation service chain? This chapter outlines community triggering strategies, tools, and tactics that have been used to galvanize action along the sanitation chain. It includes ideas of ways to get commitments and actions from different stakeholders and gives guidance on community-led action planning.

Keywords: Triggering, institutional advocacy, triggering strategy, sanitation service chain, community-led action planning

Key messages

- U-CLTS triggering involves mobilizing the community through a process of analysing their own sanitation situation. This helps citizens to confront dangerous practices and as a result galvanizes community-led action to address local sanitation challenges.
- Triggering should motivate both individual and collective action within the community.
- Both communities and duty-bearers should feed into a planning process that sets out an agenda for action.
- Advocating institutions by confronting them with the realities of urban sanitation and mobilizing commitment to respond to citizens' urban sanitation demands can create the basis for institutional and citizen accountability for better urban sanitation services.

Purpose of U-CLTS triggering

Triggering is a process of igniting passion that is channelled into building the commitment of individuals, groups, or/and institutions to take individual and collective action to address poor sanitation challenges facing their urban communities across the sanitation service chain. The aim of combined community

http://dx.doi.org/10.3362/9781780447360.003

and institutional action is to develop a shared realistic plan to achieve a shit-free environment.

This chapter focuses on three elements:

- *Community triggering.* Community triggering in an urban area taps into the disgust, frustration, and even anger that people feel about their sanitation context. This has the power to ignite them to take collective action and subsequently experience concurrent positive emotions such as pride, self-respect, and dignity.
- *Community-led action planning.* This may include making commitments for local toilet construction, improvement, and/or maintenance by community members and/or devising a strategy to engage with other relevant stakeholders in order to address the aspects of the sanitation chain for which they are responsible. The planning process should include the allocation of tasks, clear dates for completion, and strategies for monitoring progress.
- *Institutional advocacy.* Relationships with some institutional actors should have been established already – with the municipal government, for example – and these actors should be involved in facilitating the whole U-CLTS process. Additional advocacy efforts are likely to be needed for other duty-bearers who can be triggered to realize that their inaction (or perhaps their inappropriate action) is causing avoidable sickness and death, with significant public health, social, and economic consequences. Exposing them to the realities of the sanitation context in poor communities can trigger them into action or into allocating necessary funding, if such funding exists. In any case, they should then be facilitated to plan actions to address challenges in the areas of sanitation for which they are responsible, whether through their own action-planning process or by contributing to the community action planning and strengthening their own planning processes.

When planning the triggering process in an urban area it is important to think about the interplay between mobilizing the community and engaging institutions through respective triggering processes. They do not necessarily take place in a linear manner. Evidence from community triggering and the participation of mobilized community members can be effective tools for triggering institutional actors. The participation of institutional stakeholders in community triggering can also have an impact by demonstrating that the issue is being taken seriously and that there is a commitment to support community action. Triggering institutional actors should be brought into the community action planning process. U-CLTS and community actions will need to be integrated into existing Sanitation Master Plans or City Master Plans (see Chapter 3 section 'Institutional advocacy and action planning').

The tools and tactics to be used during community triggering, institutional advocacy, and action planning will be based on your particular urban typology and the information gathered in the assessment and preparation phase.

Community triggering

Community triggering in an urban context broadly shares the same aims and strategy as triggering in a rural context. In rural areas, triggering relies on a process of bringing about a realization that, due to OD, people are eating one another's shit, and that sense of disgust promptly ignites a desire to act. People in urban areas tend to be more aware of the health and well-being consequences of poor sanitation. The density of the population and buildings means that there are far fewer areas to comfortably practise OD, and therefore privacy is an important motivator. Poorly maintained, unclean, or overflowing toilets are highly unpleasant, and often unsafe to use. In many urban areas, the negative experience of using highly unsanitary facilities can impact hugely on day-to-day well-being. Given this context, the triggering may ignite other emotions such as anger and frustration in relation to various failures along the sanitation chain. The important outcome is channelling the emotion into motivation for action.

A range of tools are used for urban triggering: namely, sanitation mapping; calculation of shit; calculation of medical expenses; transect walk; and demonstration of faecal oral transmission using shit and water. The variations in how they can be used in an urban context are detailed below. All these tools are described in detail in the *Handbook on CLTS* (Kar with Chambers, 2008); what follows are ways in which they have been adapted to urban environments.

There are two key issues that should be considered in planning an urban triggering:

- the unit of community triggering; and
- the triggering strategy.

The unit of community triggering

Towns and cities are made up of large and diverse communities of people. While urban areas may be broken down into administrative units, these may still be too large (in terms of population) for triggering in a single event, requiring further subdivision into smaller triggering units. The population within those units may be heterogeneous in terms of: their length of time living in the community; culture, religion and even language; migrant or transient populations not knowing one another well; and a mix of landlords and tenants with difficult power dynamics.

These factors mean that the unit of triggering is not always obvious, and you may need to consider new and creative ways of defining 'community' in the urban context. The lack of social cohesion found in some urban settings can discourage people from coming together in community meetings and from feeling inspired to work together towards a shared common goal (safely managed sanitation). Transient members, such as street sleepers and short-term migrant labourers, may well miss any triggering events despite the best efforts to time them for maximum effect.

It is important to consider all these issues when choosing the triggering units. Work done during assessment and preparation will have provided you with information to make appropriate decisions (see Chapter 2 'Situation analysis', 'Stakeholder analysis and identifying key partners', and 'Preparing to enter the community'). It may be necessary to hold multiple triggering events at different sites and at different times of day, for example within large compounds or in streets that cut through a neighbourhood. 'Mob triggering' (see 'Triggering strategy' below) may also be held in marketplaces, bus stations, parks, etc. to catch traders, shoppers, and passers-by. It is also important to ensure that those typically excluded (female-headed households, the elderly, disabled, etc.) are able to participate; in some circumstances separate triggerings for vulnerable groups may be needed.

Triggering strategy

An additional challenge in mobilizing people for triggering in urban areas is that people tend to have much busier lives. Livelihoods tend to involve waged labour, long hours of street or market selling, and people travelling to different locations within a town or city, often working long shifts. Men and women often both work outside the home. Messages spread between neighbourhoods, which can affect the power of triggering tools. Finding a suitable time when a majority of people can participate in triggering is key. This is an issue to be explored during assessment and preparation (Chapter 2), to ensure that the day of the week, time of day, location, etc. are suitable in order to reach the desired audience. In some cases, it has been helpful to hold the triggering events at weekends, in the evenings, on public holidays, market days, or other celebrations such as World Toilet Day. Again, multiple events will be needed to mobilize the whole population. Different strategies may need to be considered to attract and maintain attention during the triggering: for example, drumming, loudhailers, singing, etc. Street theatre groups have successfully been used to draw an initial crowd. The triggering tools can then be interspersed between scenes in a creative way to ensure that people's attention is held.

Start triggering with communities with favourable conditions (often relatively small and homogeneous, with a record of diarrhoeal sickness) and then build on success. Firstly, use the information collected during the assessment and preparation stage to identify groups of people who could be triggered together. This could be, for example, church groups, market traders, restaurant owners, or landlords. These groups can then be called together and triggered using the different tools explained below.

STAGE 2: U-CLTS TRIGGERING AND INSTITUTIONAL ADVOCACY   47

TOOL 3.1 – Sanitation street theatre

What is it?	Live street theatre involves loud and engaging performances used to drum up and maintain interest
Why use it?	Street theatre is increasingly being employed in both rural and urban areas as a triggering tool in itself, but also as a means to attract attention and bring people together for the purposes of carrying out other triggering tools. Performances can be designed around faecal pollution, shit-free environments, and other U-CLTS-related themes. It can also be used to maintain audience participation if people are becoming bored or distracted by other things.
How to use it	Sanitation street theatre can consist of a short play or series of sketches, usually with comic elements: e.g. about people who fall sick through poor sanitation, or families who will not allow their children to marry into a household without a sanitary toilet. A local troupe can be engaged for this purpose and given ideas and direction to develop a suitable performance.
	Performance can be used to obtain media coverage. Photographs taken by the troupe or local photographers may appear in local newspapers with stories about the event. Good performances can be videoed and shared again later.
When would you use it?	Before the start of a triggering event with the triggering starting immediately afterwards and throughout where necessary.
Related case studies	Case Study 4: Gulariya, Nepal.

TACTIC 3.1 – Triggering homogeneous groups

What is it?	When triggering groups are homogeneous and there are relatively high levels of social capital between them.
Why use it?	Homogeneous groups are likely to have stronger social ties, making it easier to develop agreement among participants, and there is more chance that they will work together.
How to use it	Firstly, use the information collected during the assessment and preparation stage to identify groups of people who could be triggered together. These could be, for example, church/mosque groups, market traders, restaurant owners, or landlords.
	These groups can then be called together and triggered using the different tools explained below.
When would you use it?	As a strategy for triggering.
Related case studies	Case Study 12: Nakuru, Kenya.

> **Example 3.1 – Triggering homogeneous groups**
>
> In Rosso, Mauritania, triggering was done by neighbourhood as well as by homogeneous groups such as market merchants, fishermen, livestock salesmen, and religious school students. Triggering at different sites was conducted almost simultaneously and the city was treated as an overall unit. Competition between the different sub-units was encouraged. The process led to close to 32,000 people now living in an ODF environment.
>
> *Source:* Myers et al., 2016.

TACTIC 3.2 – Mob triggering

What is it?	Mob triggering is when large numbers of facilitators trigger different parts of the neighbourhood or town in unison, engaging the entire urban centre.
Why use it?	It enables triggerings to occur simultaneously across a wide area, which means that messages are not diluted. This helps maximize the shock and impact of the U-CLTS triggering process. It can also help maintain momentum and competition between different clusters.
How to use it	A large group of facilitators enter a city, town, or neighbourhood and trigger different clusters within a given area at the same time. Each cluster is helped to develop an action plan and competition between the different clusters is encouraged.
When would you use it?	As a strategy for triggering.
Related case studies	Case Study 10: Logo, Nigeria.

> **Example 3.2 – Mob triggering**
>
> Mob triggering has been used by United Purpose as part of a Global Sanitation Fund-supported programme in Nigeria. In Abeda Town, 16 teams of U-CLTS facilitators were each allocated one neighbourhood and all triggering was conducted at the same time. The effect of this was that more than half of this small town (1,025 households in total) was triggered on the same day and at around the same time. Actions were agreed, with each cluster competing to be the first to become ODF.
>
> *Source:* Case Study 10: Logo, Nigeria.

TACTIC 3.3 – Plot/compound triggering

What is it?	Triggering of compounds where multiple families reside and often share a toilet.
Why use it?	It can help ensure that those who were not in attendance are also reached. It can also help demonstrate small, doable household-led actions.
How to use it	Plot or compound triggering uses the same tools as community/neighbourhood triggering, but with fewer people. Facilitators enter compounds or plots where multiple households reside and conduct a mini triggering at the household level.
	Households are taken to the toilets they use on the compound, if they exist, rather than to OD sites, which is what you see in community-wide triggering events.
	Ensure that a plot/compound-level action plan is developed before leaving.
When would you use it?	After community triggering events as a follow-up activity with individual compounds or plots.
Related case studies	Case Study 5: Hawassa, Ethiopia.
	Case Study 11: Mathare 10, Nairobi, Kenya.

Example 3.3 – Compound triggering

In Hawassa, Ethiopia, Plan International conducted household/compound triggering sessions as a follow-up to community triggering. Each compound was visited and households living on the compound were brought together for a smaller triggering event. Pathways for faecal contamination were demonstrated with water, bread/biscuits, and kitchen utensils. Households were also taken to toilets in the same way that communities in rural areas are taken to OD sites.

Source: Case Study 5: Hawassa, Ethiopia; Myers, 2016.

Triggering tools

Most of the triggering tools for U-CLTS are based on those used in a rural context but have been adapted for use in an urban area. Suggestions are provided within tools below. However, facilitators should use their own best judgement and imagination to ensure that the tools are fit for purpose. It is suggested that the triggering process starts with mapping, although this is not essential. The tools should be used flexibly, in a logical order, so that they build on discussions that are initiated by the community. Once the community is 'triggered' (see Chapter 3 section 'U-CLTS ignition'), there may not be a need to continue through the remainder of the tools.

Tip 3.1 – Triggering for what?

Triggering in urban environments is not just for households to be galvanized to build toilets but to identify what actions are in their power to take along the sanitation chain. These could include:

- connecting to existing infrastructure or paying for existing services;
- maintaining and operating community toilets;
- stopping bad FSM practices such as emptying toilets during heavy rains;
- advocating for improved services;
- developing community by-laws; and
- cleaning up filthy communal areas.

The feasible options need to be identified in the assessment and preparation phase. However, this does not mean that ideas need to be imposed on communities, but that the programme/project/intervention team has some ideas about what could work.

Tip 3.2 – Considering vulnerability

The triggering process can be used to highlight a shared problem and gain commitment to work towards a common goal. **U-CLTS tools should never involve personally shaming people or shaming groups of already vulnerable or marginalized people**.

TOOL 3.2 – Sanitation mapping

What is it?	A tool for getting all community members involved in a practical and visual analysis of the community's sanitation situation.
How to use it	Community members identify a large open area of ground where the map can be drawn. If space is lacking in urban areas, other approaches to mapping may need to be sought (e.g. using an expanse of wall with chalks or covered in flip-chart paper). Alternatively, existing maps can be printed and information can be transferred onto them. Geographic information systems (GIS)

programmes can be valuable in this respect as different layers of information can be built up in a computerized model (see Example 3.4).

During the mapping exercise, all households are invited to locate themselves on the map, and indicate where they shit. Public and private toilets can be marked, perhaps with details about whether they are currently usable. Are there any overflow pipes? Where do they drain into? Who empties the latrines? Where does the faecal waste go? Areas used for OD or dumping will also become apparent. As with OD hotspots, a community typically knows about disposal hotspots or vacuum tankers, if there are any.

Ask questions probing the meaning and implications of what has been shown. The map can capture features such as quality and usage of toilets, solid waste dumping sites, open drains, sanitation in public places (markets, bus stations), etc.

The map should be a means to help the community get a visual understanding of the sanitation situation, not an end in itself. Ask people to trace the flow of shit from places of unsafe containment, emptying, and transportation to water bodies, resulting in their contamination – including flows coming from outside a given settlement. Draw attention to how far some people have to walk to defecate and at what times of day. Ask if there are any safety issues?

A map made on the ground can later be transferred onto paper, illustrating which households have latrines and which do not. It can then be displayed in a public place and used as a basis for monitoring change. GIS maps also need to be made available to people in an accessible format in which the information is easy to understand. The sanitation map can also form the basis of a faecal waste/shit-flow diagram to which other stakeholders can also contribute (see Chapter 3 section 'Institutional advocacy tools and tactics').

Further guidance	Kar with Chambers, 2008, http://www.communityledtotalsanitation.org/resource/handbook-community-led-total-sanitation
	Lundine et al., 2012, https://www.researchgate.net/publication/259751234
	Pasteur and Prabhakaran, 2015, www.communityledtotalsanitation.org/sites/communityledtotalsanitation.org/files/PracticalAction_LessonsOnUrbanCLTSNakuruKenya_Apr2015.pdf

> **Example 3.4 – GIS mapping**
>
> Global information systems (GIS) are software and tools for creating digital maps using geographical data. Many organizations invest in creating GIS maps that can then be viewed digitally or printed out. Using GIS, it is possible to map OD and sludge-dumping hotspots, public toilets (both functioning and defunct), service providers, and existing sanitation infrastructure (i.e. sewers, disposal facilities, etc.). These maps can then be used for different ends such as community triggering, getting institutional buy-in, and monitoring.
>
> In Nakuru, these maps were used to trigger landlords to take action. Data on coverage and the incidence of OD was collected by Community Health Volunteers who visited all the plots, and was then mapped. Landlords were then shown the maps, which highlighted inadequate coverage and areas with particularly high OD.
>
> *Source*: Pasteur and Prabhakaran, 2015.

TOOL 3.3 – Shit calculation

What is it?	This tool involves calculating the amount of shit produced by the community over a period of time.
Why use it?	Calculating the amount of faeces produced helps illustrate the magnitude of the sanitation problem and the effects it is having.
How to use it	The crowd is asked to estimate the approximate weight of one shit. They then estimate the quantity of shit each household might produce each day. This is multiplied by the number of households in the locality. A daily figure can be multiplied to know how much shit is produced per week, per month, or per year. The calculation should be done on a flip chart for all to see. The quantities can add up to a matter of tonnes, which may surprise the community. The facilitator need not be concerned with exact amounts but just an approximation.
	The calculations of quantities of shit produced by the community should lead into further questions and discussions: for example, where does all the shit go? How much is managed unsafely? How much (if any) is entering the community? What are the possible effects of having so much shit in close proximity to so many people? What are the implications for human health? What happens when the pits fill up? This can lead on to a discussion of faecal–oral transmission routes, or the calculation of medical expenses (see Tools 3.7 and 3.10).
Further guidance/ related case studies	Case Study 5: Hawassa, Ethiopia. Case Study 4: Gulariya, Nepal. Kar with Chambers, 2008, http://www.communityledtotalsanitation.org/resource/handbook-community-led-total-sanitation

TOOL 3.4 – Household medical expenses calculation

What is it?	Calculating medical expenses spent on waterborne disease helps illustrate the direct impact of the sanitation problem on the household economy.
Why use it?	People calculate how much money they spend on average per month on medical treatment for preventable diseases for both adults and children in the household. The figures are multiplied to produce a total household expenditure for the year. This can be multiplied to produce an annual figure for the whole neighbourhood. Could this expenditure be prevented?
How to use it	Ask people how much they spend on average per month on consultations and medicine for preventable diseases such as diarrhoea, dysentery, cholera, etc. They should include expenses incurred for the whole household – adults and children. Include transport to clinics and hospitals. This can be multiplied to produce an annual figure for the whole community or neighbourhood, per month and then per year. The calculation should be done on a flip chart for all to see. It is typically a shocking total.
	This could be the starting point for further discussion. Which families spend the most? Do they live close to the dirtiest neighbourhood? Are people so well off that they can afford to spend so much? Do any poor families borrow money for emergency treatment of diarrhoea for any family member? Was it easy to borrow money and repay it? Who lends money for emergency treatment and at what rate of interest? Finally, how could this expenditure be prevented?
	It is useful to use this tool straight after the shit calculation.
	Other expenses that result from not having a toilet at home can also be discussed, such as the costs of being reliant on pay-per-use toilets.
Further guidance/ related case studies	Case Study 5: Hawassa, Ethiopia. Kar with Chambers, 2008, http://www.communityledtotal sanitation.org/resource/handbook-community-led-total-sanitation

TOOL 3.5 – Transect walk

What is it?	A transect walk involves walking with people through the community, observing, asking questions, and listening.
Why use it?	Transect walks are an important triggering tool. The embarrassment experienced during this walk often results in an immediate desire to stop unsafe sanitation practices and to clean up filthy areas. Even though everyone sees the dirt and shit every day, they only seem to wake up to the problem when they focus on it and analyse the situation in detail.
How to use it	A transect walk should purposefully include areas of: • OD; • fixed-point OD (i.e. toilets where there is exposed shit or that are not fly-proof); • hanging toilets or flying toilets; • overflowing latrines; • toilet outlets discharging directly into open drains; and • indiscriminate dumping of human waste either produced within the community or entering from somewhere else. It is important to stop in the most unpleasant areas (of OD, poorly maintained toilets, or polluted environments) and spend time there asking questions while inhaling the unpleasant smell and taking in the unpleasant sights. If people try to move on, insist on staying there. Facilitators can take pictures and video clips on their phones. Experiencing the disgusting sight and smell in this new way, accompanied by a visitor to the community, is a key factor that triggers mobilization. In many urban settlements, people often live in compounds and can feel uncomfortable about strangers walking through. It is important to be aware of this. Triggering at the compound level rather than community level may be appropriate in these circumstances. The transect walk is a good opportunity to use the shit and water tool (see Tool 3.6 – shit and water).
Further guidance/ related case studies	Case Study 5: Hawassa, Ethiopia. Kar with Chambers, 2008, http://www.communityledtotalsanitation.org/resource/handbook-community-led-total-sanitation

Tip 3.3 – Transect walks

Experience is varied with transect walks in urban areas. Programmes in Madagascar and Indonesia have avoided them as it was a struggle to walk with large groups of people through narrow lanes, and they found that people got distracted and wandered off, impeding the triggering process. Whether or not they are used will depend on whether they are apposite in a particular context.

This is something to consider before you begin triggering activities.

TOOL 3.6 – Shit and water

What is it?	This is a tool for demonstrating a faecal–oral transmission route.
Why use it?	It can ignite a strong sense of disgust at the realization that people might be drinking one another's shit. It can lead to a discussion of other transmission routes that ultimately affect human health.
How to use it	Ask for a glass or a bottle of drinking water. When the glass of water is brought, offer it to someone and ask if they could drink it. Next, pull a hair from your head and touch it on some shit on the ground so that everyone can see. Now dip the hair in the glass of water and ask if they can see anything in the glass of water. Next, offer the glass of water to several different people in the gathering and ask them to drink it. No one will want to drink that water. Ask why they refuse it. They will answer that it contains shit. Now ask if flies could pick up more or less shit than your hair could. Ask what happens when flies sit on their or their children's food or plate. This is often a key ignition moment.
Further guidance	Kar with Chambers, 2008, http://www.communityledtotalsanitation.org/resource/handbook-community-led-total-sanitation

TOOL 3.7 – Faecal–oral contamination routes

What is it?	An opportunity for discussion of the different ways in which shit moves around the community, enters the household, and might be ingested by people.
How to use it	This discussion might take place during mapping once people have marked hotspots of unsafe faecal management. Ask where all that shit goes. As people answer that it is washed away by the rain, or enters drains or rivers, draw a picture of a lump of shit and put it on the ground. Put cards and markers near it.
	Ask people to pick up the cards and draw or write the different agents or pathways that bring shit into the home: for example, flies, storm-water drains, floodwater, fruit and vegetables grown in urban environments, rainwater, wind, hoofs of domestic animals, chickens

that eat shit or have it on their feet and wings, dogs that eat shit or have it on their paws or bodies, shit-smeared ropes (e.g. used for tethering animals), bicycle tyres, shoes, children's toys, footballs, windblown waste plastic, contaminated water, etc.

Then ask how the shit then gets into the mouth: for example, on hands, fingernails, flies on food, fruit and vegetables that have fallen on or been in contact with shit and not been washed, utensils washed in contaminated water, dogs licking people, toys or balls that have been in drains, children playing in contaminated river or drain water and entering the home, etc. You should never suggest the pathway of contamination. Let people discuss, identify, and draw/write.

Further guidance	Kar with Chambers, 2008, http://www.communityledtotalsanitation.org/resource/handbook-community-led-total-sanitation

TOOL 3.8 – Participatory video/photography

What is it?	Participatory video is a set of techniques to involve a group or community in taking their own photographs or creating their own films.
Why use it?	The idea behind this is that making a video and taking photographs can be easy and accessible and are great ways of bringing people together to explore issues, voice concerns, or simply be creative and tell stories.
	The filmmaking/photography process can enable participants to take action to solve their own problems, or to communicate their needs and ideas to decision-makers.
How to use it	The easiest way of doing it is by asking community members to use their own mobile phones to take photos and videos of bad sanitation practices. These could include leaking pipes, flying toilets, and hand toilets as well as evidence of OD.
	These images can then be shared with others.
	It is important not to show photos or videos of people defecating as this can cause embarrassment and violate human rights.
When would you use it?	It can be used as an effective tool during the assessment and preparation stage, in triggering, or to maintain momentum.
Further guidance/ related case studies	Case Study 4: Gulariya, Nepal.
	Case Study 14: Ribaué and Rapale, Mozambique.
	Case Study 8: IUWASH, Indonesia.
	IUWASH, 2015, https://www.iuwashplus.or.id/cms/wp-content/uploads/2017/04/Guide-to-Urban-Sanitation-Promotion-EN.pdf

STAGE 2: U-CLTS TRIGGERING AND INSTITUTIONAL ADVOCACY

> **Example 3.5 – Triggering for connecting to existing infrastructure**
>
> Part of the Indonesia Urban Water, Sanitation, and Hygiene (IUWASH) programme focused on improving FSM systems, getting communities to connect existing latrines to sewers, or building septic tanks rather than having waste draining into rivers, canals, and gutters. They found that transect walks were unsuccessful. Instead, they asked community members to walk around the neighbourhood and use their mobile phones to take photos of bad FSM practices. These photos were then shown in community meetings.
>
> *Source*: Case Study 8: IUWASH, Indonesia; IUWASH, 2015.

TOOL 3.9 – Analysing water contamination

What is it?	Communities can be triggered by either involving them in water testing or sharing the results of water tests.
Why use it?	Where there might be an assumption that piped or well water is clean, this can be the starting point for a discussion around how poor sanitation is contaminating the water supply.
How to use it	This could be done in many ways and innovation is encouraged.
	The hydrogen sulphate test requires the purchase and distribution of field testing kits. Water from wells and piped water is then tested by community members to see if it is contaminated with faecal matter. Later that day or the following day, community members are asked to present the results in a public forum.
	Another option is to post water quality data in a public place where everyone can see and use it as a discussion point.
When would you use it?	Triggering.
Further guidance/ related case studies	Case Study 9: Kabwe, Zambia.
	Myers, 2016, http://www.communityledtotalsanitation.org/sites/communityledtotalsanitation.org/files/Urban_CLTS_Plan.pdf

> **Example 3.6 – Using water contamination data**
>
> In Nala, Nepal, as part of a Community-Led Urban Environmental Sanitation programme, data about the extent of water contamination at each of the key water sources around the community was posted on a public sign board, both shocking participants and motivating them to take action.
>
> *Source*: Myers et al., 2016.

U-CLTS ignition

U-CLTS 'ignition' refers to the moment when participants in the triggering process start to express an emotional response to the issues raised by the U-CLTS triggering tools and ensuing discussion. They may feel disgust, frustration, or even anger about the sanitation situation they are experiencing. This is the moment to channel those emotions towards coming up with potential collective actions for change and agreements about ways forward. It is important when using the above tools to be alert for this moment. Once people appear moved towards taking action there is no need to continue with other tools. It is then time to mobilize people's commitment to take direct action in the areas where they can – i.e. stopping any OD, building or upgrading and repairing toilets, cleaning up their existing communal/shared toilets and managing them better, hygienically emptying full pits, connecting houses to a sewer, etc.

At the ignition moment, encourage people to suggest ways in which they could address sanitation issues that they may currently consider to be beyond their control. To support this process you can share examples of where and how change has happened elsewhere. It is important to be prepared for this moment, and already have some ideas about how the community may be able to solve their sanitation problems and also how they can be supported to implement their own actions and/or claim their right to sanitation via duty-bearers, including landlords, municipal government, service providers, etc. Impress on them the fact that, without their commitment and determination, nothing is likely to happen. They need to organize themselves to take action. You have not come to do it for them.

Creating a comprehensive plan to address the complexity of the sanitation situation will require more time. Identify those Natural Leaders (see below) who are emerging from the discussion and suggest that they organize a further meeting at which they will be supported to develop an action plan and to work alongside the community, project partners, and other stakeholders to address the concerns raised during the triggering. Encourage them to take a leadership role, setting a date and suggesting a location to meet among themselves as well as with local government and utilities representatives.

Natural Leaders

'Natural Leader' is a term used to describe local champions who are vocal in the triggering process and are determined to take action to change the current sanitation situation. They may already have a significant role in the community, for example as a Community Health Volunteer or local leader, or they may simply emerge as an impassioned individual. It is important that leadership of any initiative is grounded within the community rather than driven from outside. This will contribute significantly to local ownership and sustainability.

Natural Leaders can be nurtured immediately by acknowledging their comments within the triggering process, asking them to explain to the rest of those present why they are so passionate about the issue of sanitation, encouraging the crowd to applaud their positive comments, or backing up their comments with further support. Over time, Natural Leaders can be supported with encouragement, training, materials, etc. that will help them function as effectively as possible in working with the wider community to plan and implement relevant actions.

It is important to strive for a gender balance and have equal numbers of male and female Natural Leaders.

Community-led action planning processes

The objective of this stage is to develop an action plan for the community to:

- take action themselves to improve their sanitation situation; and
- engage with wider stakeholders to ensure that they take appropriate action to address sanitation challenges that locals cannot act on alone.

The planning process should be based on widespread participation and commitment from the community. It can be developed by a group of Natural Leaders, a sanitation committee that forms after a triggering event, or with a wider group of people. It should also engage and involve other relevant stakeholders with responsibilities for delivering aspects of sanitation that cannot be achieved by the community. The process will require careful facilitation to ensure that the community is able to drive the process but that other stakeholders can also make relevant commitments.

Timelines for this process need to be thought through on a case-by-case basis. It is unlikely that a community triggering will lead directly into an action planning process; however, it will be important that planning occurs as soon as possible to keep momentum.

Actions within the community can serve as 'quick wins' that mobilize more people and motivate them to engage in other stakeholder forums and to bring about wider change. They might include any of the following depending on the local context: constructing latrines; cleaning up or emptying existing facilities; connecting to existing infrastructure such as sewers or paying for services; ceasing OD; and/or cleaning up former OD sites. They may also include community advocacy to responsible agencies, or the community joining with a sanitation initiative in another part of the town, or becoming a 'pilot site' for an FSM trial. It is important to fully engage people and maintain momentum for action within households, larger compounds, and the wider community. Actions that can be taken by both the community and wider stakeholders are detailed in Chapter 4.

Facilitators of the U-CLTS process should develop a strategy to guide communities, along with public - and private-sector stakeholders, towards collaboratively developing a community-led stakeholder action plan. Facilitation should be sensitive to the power dynamics that might exist between the different stakeholders. Key elements of this strategy should include the following:

1. Draw on studies undertaken in the assessment and preparation stage as well as the findings of the community triggering exercises to identify issues, gaps in services, and relevant stakeholders and related projects and programmes.
2. Assess what actions can be taken by the community and what actions will need support from others (see Chapter 4). Commitments within City Sanitation Plans may provide a useful means of leveraging participation and action by public, NGO, and private stakeholders.
3. Bring key community representatives together with relevant public, NGO, and private-sector actors in a number of collaborative planning events. A working group may be formed of community representatives and other stakeholders who are key to the success of the process. Meetings may require external facilitation to maintain a fair power balance.
4. Develop an aspirational but realistic vision of a clean city neighbourhood that both community and wider stakeholders are committed to, with a clear, shared understanding of how it will be achieved. It may be useful to find a way to capture and publicize stakeholders' commitment: for example, in the form of a video or publicly signed agreement that can be used to hold all to account during implementation.
5. Carry out a process of validation and prioritization of those issues raised by the community and those issues emerging from wider analysis of the sanitation context, including issues proposed by wider stakeholders. This process should be led by the community and should aim to identify priority issues for incorporation in the plan.
6. The plan should consider phased implementation. Look at what things can be tackled relatively easily to establish some quick wins before moving on to more challenging issues. For example, start with safe containment before moving on to safe emptying and disposal.
7. Ensure that all aspects of the plan are fully budgeted. Financial support may come from landlords, households, the municipal government, national government, or NGO programmes, etc. Financial commitments should be closely monitored to ensure that they are realized.
8. Develop a realistic timeline with easy-to-measure indicators and targets which the community and other stakeholders can work towards

achieving: for example, reducing the number of OD hotspots or increasing the number of houses with an improved latrine. Develop a range of tools for monitoring and measures for addressing delays (see Chapter 5).
9. Incorporate moments for reflection, learning, and celebrating successes during implementation of the community-led action plan (see Chapter 5). This can help to ensure that enthusiasm is sustained, good relationships are maintained, and relevant lessons are learned during what may be a lengthy process of implementation.

The preparation required for action to achieve wider changes and investments in the later stages of the sanitation service chain will be a more complex process of analysis and planning, and will need to be led at the institutional level.

TOOL 3.10 – Scenario planning

What is it?	Scenario planning is an alternative planning tool and is intended to make stakeholders think about possible futures, as well as stimulate creative thinking. It motivates people to challenge the status quo by asking 'What if?'
Why use it?	This has been used in planning and informing investment decisions in public health. Scenarios are a useful tool to encourage discussion on a shared issue. Scenarios can be suggested by research or implementation teams or they can be created in a participatory process by community members.
How to use it	This kind of planning, informed by your situation analysis or baseline, will help outline how you intend to deliver your programme (aims, objectives, activities, indicators, outputs, outcomes, impact, budget, and resources) in various scenarios. It aims to help overcome or solve problems identified in the situation analysis or baseline. Scenario planning helps to mitigate risks and ensure that approaches work towards access and use of services by all.
	It will help to plan carefully to address barriers to improved sanitation for all. When combined with the situation analysis, it should inform a programme plan. It should also be used to help implementers assess what options are feasible for a particular area. If no practical options are identified, a U-CLTS approach may not be appropriate.
	It can be conducted in many ways with different levels of community involvement.
	In Hoang Tay Commune, in Hanam Province, a peri-urban community in Vietnam, participants constructed scenarios describing what their commune would look like in 10 years if the sanitation situation remained unchanged. They then identified next steps. Scenario planning was used to identify problem-solving options and address priority issues at the commune level. The focal issue was designing a clean water and sanitation system (upgrading the drainage system,

	waste collection, and treatment) with community contributions. Focus group discussions were used to construct scenarios and identify options. One month of scoping and household visits in between the focus group meetings was used to help understand and contextualize the data collected from the focus groups.
When would you use it?	As a community action planning exercise.
Further guidance	Nguyen et al., 2014, http://doi:10.3402/gha.v7.24482

TOOL 3.11 – Ranking and prioritization tool

What is it?	Different methods may be used for ranking and/or prioritizing different issues raised in community analysis and the situation analysis in order to decide how and when they are addressed in the action plan.
Why use it?	This tool allows different stakeholders to have an input in the prioritization of issues, which could otherwise be co-opted by more vocal or powerful participants in the process.
How to use it	Ranking and prioritization can happen in a number of ways. They can be facilitated in small focus group discussions so that there is an opportunity for discussion of the issues before reaching a collective decision. The outcomes of different focus groups would then need to be collated in a plenary forum. Options can also be ranked through either a public or a private voting system, whereby each participant in the process can vote for their most favoured element(s) for inclusion.
Further guidance	Lüthi et al., 2011b, http://www.eawag.ch/fileadmin/Domain1/Abteilungen/sandec/schwerpunkte/sesp/CLUES/CLUES_Guidelines.pdf

> **Box 3.1 Guides for urban sanitation planning**
>
> The following references may be helpful in designing your community-led urban sanitation planning process:
>
> Lüthi, C., Morel, A., Tilley, E. and Ulrich, L. (2011b) *Community-Led Urban Environmental Sanitation: CLUES. A Complete Guide for Decision Makers with 30 Tools*, Eawag, UN Habitat, and WSSCC, Dübendorf, Switzerland, http://www.eawag.ch/fileadmin/Domain1/Abteilungen/sandec/schwerpunkte/sesp/CLUES/CLUES_Guidelines.pdf [accessed 25 February 2018].
>
> WaterAid (2016) *A Tale of Clean Cities: Insights for Planning Urban Sanitation from Ghana, India and the Philippines*, synthesis and full reports), WaterAid, London.

Institutional advocacy and action planning

Expecting communities to take full control of addressing their poor sanitation situation is unrealistic. This is particularly true in urban areas. While the U-CLTS process is community-led, it is not communities alone that should act and community action plans will need to be supported by other stakeholders. They will also need to be incorporated into existing or future plans (see Table 3.16 Tool – City Sanitation Plans or Sanitation Master Plans).

Table 3.1 Actions likely to be needed by each stakeholder group

Stakeholder	Focus for stakeholder action
Representatives of municipal government or service delivery organizations	• Investment in sanitation within communities, e.g. sewer connections, toilets in public spaces, markets, hospitals, schools, etc. • Uptake/scaling-up of U-CLTS approach.
Private sector	• Landlords to negotiate options for appropriate sanitation facilities for tenants. • Entrepreneurs to meet the market demand for more affordable sanitation hardware. • Extractors of faecal sludge to find ways to reach low-income areas.
Political and non-political leaders or groups	• Mobilization for lobbying of municipal government.

TOOL 3.12 – City Sanitation Plans or Sanitation Master Plans

What is it?	City Sanitation Plans (also known as Sanitation Master Plans) are guidance documents for local authorities to help them prioritize and organize the delivery of sanitation services. The plans may have a 10-year or longer horizon with short-, medium-, and long-term sanitation activities.
	The plans may comprise: household sanitation, institutional and public sanitation, solid waste management, hygiene behaviour change, capacity development of local government/private sector, funding requirements, and short-term action plans. But they vary enormously depending on who has commissioned them, who has funded them, and their knowledge, experience, and interest.
Why use it?	U-CLTS should be incorporated into City Sanitation Plans with respect to improving the effectiveness of proposed interventions for household sanitation, institutional and public sanitation, capacity development of local government or the private sector, and funding requirements for the cost of software.

	The provision of safe sanitation infrastructure and services in urban areas is a complex endeavour that is often not systematic, particularly for non-sewered sanitation. Significant effort is needed to integrate U-CLTS into these interventions.
	Incorporating U-CLTS means that the City Sanitation Plans can improve: the pace of urban sanitation planning and interventions; the organization of sanitation services within local government; the promotion and regulation of household and institutional sanitation; the sanitation chain; and solid waste management. U-CLTS is a cost-effective and simple to implement means of achieving results. Investment in U-CLTS as part of larger sanitation interventions (sewers, FSM services, etc.) could potentially improve the effectiveness and sustainability of services.
How to use it	The development of guidance documents should be led by municipal governments. They should set out the short-, medium- and long-term goals of the town or city. The role of NGOs and development partners is to provide coaching and mentoring for government workers to carry out short-term actions.
When would you use it?	These should already exist in large urban centres. Where they do not, they can be used as a way for institutions to develop an action plan. However, developing any plans is likely to require significant time, resources, and expertise.
Further guidance/ related case studies	Case Study 14: Ribaué and Rapale, Mozambique. Thomas and Alvestegui, 2015, www.unicef.org/esaro/WASH-Field-Small-Towns-low-res.pdf

Institutional action planning will need to run alongside or be integrated into a community-led action planning process. It brings together relevant stakeholders to develop a vision and action plan to address the sanitation situation within a particular urban locality. The action planning forum should create an opportunity for institutional stakeholders to ask questions about how they can change the situation, or make their own suggestions about what they might do, and it should create a space for them to air the challenges they face. Stakeholders may be brought together in one large single forum, or as a number of forums to address particular aspects of the sanitation challenge.

Processes of advocating to institutions and action planning can be used strategically – separately or in combination – to gain the commitment of relevant stakeholders to take prompt action to address the sanitation situation in a particular locality.

It is important to be prepared for challenges that may arise and have possible responses so that these cannot shut the discussion down. For example, be prepared to address the issue of lack of finance from stakeholders, or be ready to present examples of different technology or service delivery options that have been used elsewhere. Having some key potential actions to propose to stakeholders, rather than expecting them to find all the solutions, will help avoid creating an impasse.

> **Example 3.7 – Multiple stakeholder planning event**
>
> In Mathare 10, Nairobi, Plan International Kenya organized a stakeholder event with around 100 people from the government, representatives of different geographical areas, community-based service providers, NGOs, local businesses, youth groups, women's groups, churches, etc. The participants looked at their own roles in sanitation, their strengths and weaknesses, the resources they already had at their disposal, and their relationships with other groups. The facilitators asked people what they saw as their role in the proposed initiative. This gave them a basis on which to agree a proposal for activities going forward.
>
> *Source*: Case Study 11: Mathare 10, Nairobi, Kenya.

Institutional advocacy tools and tactics

Institutional advocacy is a process of garnering support for the U-CLTS process from local institutions that are essential to achieving total sanitation but may not already be on board or fully committed. It aims to motivate a response from relevant institutional (or individual) stakeholders who have a role to play in facilitating or delivering aspects of improved sanitation services.

Key institutional stakeholders are presented with key facts about the impacts of poor sanitation in order to elicit a powerful response, which may be based on emotional, economic, social, or other motivators. By finding out how they already see their responsibilities for sanitation, you will find out if it is necessary to motivate them to see their personal responsibility for the poor sanitation situation, and to get a greater response or action. Just as the community triggering aims to provoke a sense of disgust that in turn ignites a desire to act, institutional motivating (increasing political prioritization) can also act as a 'wake-up call', enthusing and inspiring institutional actors to commit their efforts and mobilize political will to take action where they are able. It is a useful tool when buy-in is low and/or stakeholders are failing to appreciate their own role and responsibility in addressing the sanitation situation in question.

The techniques listed below can also be used to get key partners on board during the assessment and preparation phase (Chapter 2).

66 INNOVATIONS FOR URBAN SANITATION

TOOL 3.13 – Faecal waste/shit flow diagrams

What is it?	A faecal waste flow diagram – often also known as a shit flow diagram (SFD) – is a tool to understand and communicate how excreta 'flow' through a city or town. It shows how all excreta generated in a city is or is not contained as it moves from defecation to disposal or end use. An accompanying report describes the service delivery context of the city or town. SFDs offer an innovative way to engage urban stakeholders from political leaders to sanitation experts and civil society organizations in a coordinated dialogue about excreta management.
Why use it?	To identify the current situation and the key parts of the system that need to be addressed, and to mobilize support from local authorities and other key decision makers.
How to use it	A basic SFD for the target community areas may be compiled using situation analysis data collected during the assessment and preparation stage of the U-CLTS process. It is likely to be more powerful if it is completed by the community and other sanitation stakeholders in the same town or city.
	Diagrams can be further explored with community members during community-led action planning (see Chapter 3 section 'Community-led action planning processes') and during other stakeholder planning processes that form the later part of the triggering stage. Additional information may be sought through site visits to make observations and through further discussions with community representatives or additional key informants in order to complement, validate, or challenge the data collected. The diagram should form the basis for ongoing discussion, planning, action, and updating over the course of the U-CLTS intervention. The community SFD could also be a useful comparator with the city-wide SFD, if one exists.
When would you use it?	This can be used in the assessment and preparation phase, during action planning, or as an institutional advocacy tool to stimulate action and commitments by local government and mandated service providers.
Further guidance	Peal et al., 2014, https://doi.org/10.2166/washdev.2014.139 SuSanA, n.d., www.sfd.susana.org/sfd

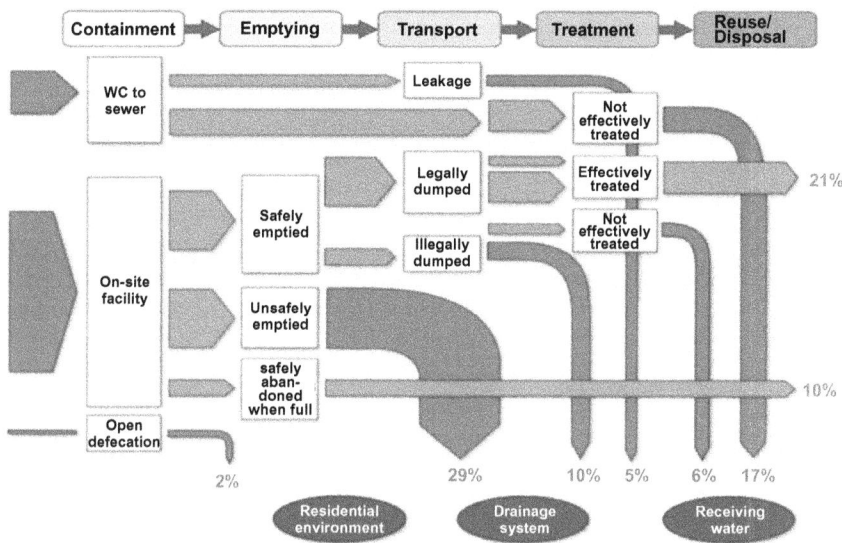

Figure 3.1 Faecal waste or shit flow diagram
Source: Blackett et al., 2014.

TACTIC 3.4 – Sharing community triggering with key stakeholders

What is it? Presenting evidence to key stakeholders about the people living with inadequate sanitation within their personal area of influence.

Why use it? This is a tool for eliciting a sense of responsibility among key stakeholders by making them more aware of the poor sanitation experience of local communities.

How to use it Evidence from the community triggering (see Chapter 3 section 'Community triggering') may be presented to key stakeholders by facilitators or by community members themselves – for example, emergent Natural Leaders – depending on which would seem to be strategically more effective. Evidence could include:

- community maps showing overall sanitation status, including the number of plots, compounds, or households with inadequate facilities and/or areas of OD;
- photographs or videos clearly illustrating unsanitary conditions that need to be addressed;
- calculations of medical expenses, illustrating the impact of poor sanitation on the household economy;
- descriptions of community members' experience of poor sanitation (these can be powerful and moving).

In some cases it may be appropriate to invite a key stakeholder to observe a triggering event first-hand. However, they should not get involved in or influence the community process.

TOOL 3.14 – Exposure visits

What is it?	Taking stakeholders to communities to expose them to good and bad sanitation contexts.
Why use it?	Exposing key stakeholders to a typically poor sanitation context may help trigger a sense of disgust and motivate them to take action. Taking them to a community that has made good progress towards a shit-free environment provides a positive motivation by illustrating what is possible.
How to use it	An exposure visit may be organized for an individual stakeholder or a group of people.

When visiting areas that have seen vast improvements it is important that stakeholders meet community members who have made those improvements and discuss how this happened.

It may be challenging to motivate senior stakeholders to leave the office for such a visit. Strategic use of events such as World Toilet Day or World Handwashing Day can create a reason for organizing the visit. |

TOOL 3.15 – Sharing the numbers

What is it?	This tool involves sharing data relating to the outcomes of poor sanitation, including health, economic, and social impacts. Information such as the numbers of people who have been affected by or have died from cholera (or other waterborne diseases) in a single year can have a big effect.
How to use it	Gather and share data relating to human, social, and economic impacts of poor sanitation in the local area. Citing the numbers of children affected by cholera can be particularly powerful. Calculations of the economic cost of illness caused by poor sanitation are also useful; for example, the WSP Country Fact Sheets for Kenya note that Nakuru County loses 978 million Kenyan shillings each year due to poor sanitation, and 50.7 per cent of children are stunted as a result of poor sanitation (WSP, 2014).

TOOL 3.16 – Landlord forums

What is it?	The landlord forum is a tool that has been used in Nakuru to motivate landlords to improve the sanitation in rental properties, typically in compounds with shared toilets.
Why use it?	To convince landlords to take action for their tenants.
How to use it	The landlord forum is essentially a form of landlord triggering. It involves bringing together all landlords within a certain area, irrespective of the standard or quality of their sanitation facilities. There would typically be around 50 landlords in such a meeting and it might last as long as three or four hours. Where a landlord is not available, a caretaker will attend in their place. Some caretakers are empowered to act on the landlord's behalf, while others will pass the information to the landlord.

The landlord forum involves the following aspects:

- Landlords are shown maps of the sanitation status in the area, including information such as the number of plots that do not have adequate sanitation facilities, the number of pits filled up, areas where waste water is found, areas of OD, etc. This is done without pinpointing the status of individual landlords' plots.
- The triggering strategy includes discussions about the health implications of poor sanitation for the people living on their plots: for example, how sickness (from diarrhoea or other waterborne diseases) reduces available income and makes rent payment more of a challenge.
- Landlords are given an explanation of the legal requirements for sanitation provision and the consequences of inadequate provision (court proceedings).
- There is discussion around tenants' rights and the fact that landlords can be sued by tenants for inadequate provision of facilities.
- The landlords are guided by the facilitators regarding details of appropriate sanitation facilities and other issues pertaining to sanitation, such as technology, sludge management, drainage, etc.
- Landlords raise their own challenges and the facilitators suggest how to overcome these themselves and advise them on the right authorities to approach to obtain approvals and to get other things done, such as getting water connections, dealing with faecal sludge, improving waste water disposal, managing solid waste, etc.
- Options for accessing finance are discussed.

	Development of an action plan is encouraged at this stage, so that there is collective commitment to change. This is built on in follow-up meetings. The landlord forum is mainly based on discussions. Traditional U-CLTS tools to trigger disgust and shame do not work in this context as many of the landlords do not live on the same plot. The role of the facilitator is key in managing the discussion so as not to create resistance. The landlords often blame the tenants for poor sanitation. However, there is heavy emphasis on the landlords' responsibility for maintaining and upgrading facilities so that tenants can keep them clean.
When would you use it?	In contexts where action is required by landlords in order to upgrade sanitation facilities in rental properties.
Further guidance/ related case studies	Case Study 12: Nakuru, Kenya. Pasteur and Prabhakaran, 2015, www.communityledtotalsanitation.org/sites/communityledtotalsanitation.org/files/PracticalAction_LessonsOnUrbanCLTSNakuruKenya_Apr2015.pdf.

Dos and don'ts for triggering, advocacy, and action planning

Table 3.2 Dos and don'ts: triggering, advocacy, and action planning

Dos	Don'ts
1. Focus on empowerment and innovation, universal access, and collective behaviour change. 2. Identify key areas of action by the community or involving external actors along the sanitation chain. Develop a collaborative strategy with inputs from communities and other relevant stakeholders. 3. Draw on good practices in urban sanitation to design actions. 4. Involve all actors in the sanitation chain. 5. Mobilize action to address safe capture and containment by community members themselves, e.g. through cleaning existing toilets, constructing additional facilities, upgrading facilities (both superstructures and containment facilities) to meet appropriate design and construction standards, improving management, installing handwashing facilities, etc.	1. Focus only on the provision of toilets – ensure that systems are in place to address all relevant aspects of the sanitation chain. Lobby or work with relevant institutions and service providers to ensure that pits and septic tanks can be emptied in a regular, safe, and affordable manner, and that sludge is appropriately transported and treated. 2. Assume that actions to address sanitation cannot be taken by communities. 3. Assume that the community is able to deliver all the necessary actions in the sanitation chain. 4. Forget the importance of affordable finance, especially for the most vulnerable. Think about the finance options to ensure that sanitation elements can be implemented: e.g. savings groups, low-cost loans, subsidised materials, etc.

Dos	Don'ts
6. Work closely with community leadership, Natural Leaders, and local entrepreneurs, as well as existing service providers, whether private, government, or parastatal. 7. Work with communities to ensure mechanisms for safe and regular emptying of pits and septic tanks. 8. Start with 'small immediate doable actions'. Community motivation will be enhanced by short-term positive achievements. 9. Ensure widespread participation (community and other stakeholders) in the analysis of market systems or technology selection. 10. Build the capacity of SMEs – e.g. for sanitation hardware supply, construction, pit emptying, solid waste collection, etc. This can improve the sustainability of services, strengthen the local economy, and provide more affordable services. 11. Identify and work with people who may be disadvantaged and need additional support or require adapted technologies. 12. Promote national regulations to ensure action to improve sanitation. However, where regulations are not relevant to low-income communities, lobby for them to be adapted.	5. Focus on hardware only – people and collective behaviour change are at the heart of achieving total urban sanitation. 6. Think about sanitation in isolation from solid and liquid waste management. Work with communities and/or other relevant institutions to put in place systems for the safe management, collection, and disposal of solid waste and waste water.

Notes for users

CHAPTER 4

Stage 3: Integrating U-CLTS across the sanitation chain

Abstract

To ensure inclusive safely managed sanitation services and create a shit-free environment in urban communities, different actions are needed across the sanitation chain – actions that can be taken by communities and actions that need to be undertaken by others. This chapter looks at both types along the different stages of the sanitation chain: safe capture and containment, safe emptying and transportation, and safe treatment, disposal, and reuse. It provides examples of what has been done in different towns and cities and provides some practical tools and tactics.

Keywords: Inclusive safely managed sanitation; sanitation chain; shit-free environment; capture and containment; emptying and transportation; treatment, disposal and reuse.

Key messages

- Creating a shit-free environment requires actions by a range of different actors across the sanitation chain.
- A U-CLTS approach emphasizes: actions to support empowerment and innovation; achieving collective behaviour change; and a focus on universal access.
- Action for total sanitation will also include aspects of solid waste and drainage management, moving beyond the human excreta sanitation chain.

Purpose of integrating U-CLTS across the sanitation chain

As mentioned in the introduction, U-CLTS is not a complete solution in itself and there is much that is still not known. This section focuses on how U-CLTS thinking can be used to tackle challenges across the sanitation chain. This is not a comprehensive list of ways to achieve safely managed sanitation and it is not based exclusively on U-CLTS programmes. What it provides are tools, tactics, ideas, and thinking for how to increase community participation in

http://dx.doi.org/10.3362/9781780447360.004

action and decision-making processes across the sanitation chain, alongside ensuring a total shit-free environment.

As part of the assessment, preparation, and triggering processes, community members and other stakeholders propose an action plan prioritizing activity to eliminate exposure to faeces in their neighbourhood. The purpose of this step is to create an enabling environment that facilitates this action, allowing people to move as fast as possible in addressing their prioritized issues. Achieving a shit-free environment in urban communities requires action across the sanitation chain, so facilitators need to consider the following:

- *Safe capture and containment.* To tackle OD hotspots, flying toilets, poorly maintained and used toilets, toilets that overflow into drains or waterways, and unused full latrines (because they cannot be emptied). Also the building, fixing, cleaning, and maintaining of shared, communal, or public toilets, ensuring increased coverage, reducing numbers sharing a toilet (limited sanitation) to reasonable levels, and increased use of safe and appropriate technologies for containment.
- *Safe emptying and transportation.* To ensure that faecal sludge is safely removed to a point where it can be treated and disposed of. An end to unhygienic manual emptying practices, open dumping of faecal sludge, flushing of pits during rainy seasons, and the opening of pits and septic tanks directly into drains.
- *Safe treatment, disposal, and possibly reuse.* To ensure that faecal waste removed from or retained in the community is safely treated or disposed of – and, wherever possible, reused.

Figure 4.1 illustrates the sanitation chain. An additional step of disposal has been included between transport and treatment. Although it often does not appear in the diagram of the sanitation chain (figure 1.1), it is common for manual pit emptiers to bury (dispose of) pit content on-site without treatment. Below the chain are actions that can be taken by communities. Above are actions that require inputs from other stakeholders. The arrow of influence is there to stress that, even though they may not have direct control, community participation in decision-making is important and the potential exists to influence decision-makers.

In addition to the human excreta chain, **associated waste streams**, including menstrual hygiene products, also need attention. Refuse – including diapers, sanitary pads or rags, household refuse, etc. – can block toilets or contaminate drains and open spaces. Disposing of rubbish in pit latrines significantly increases costs and can prevent mechanical emptying, which means that the only other option is manual emptying. These actions need to be combined with regular follow-up, as described in Chapter 5, which aims to keep energy levels high and to maintain momentum.

STAGE 3: INTEGRATING U-CLTS ACROSS THE SANITATION CHAIN

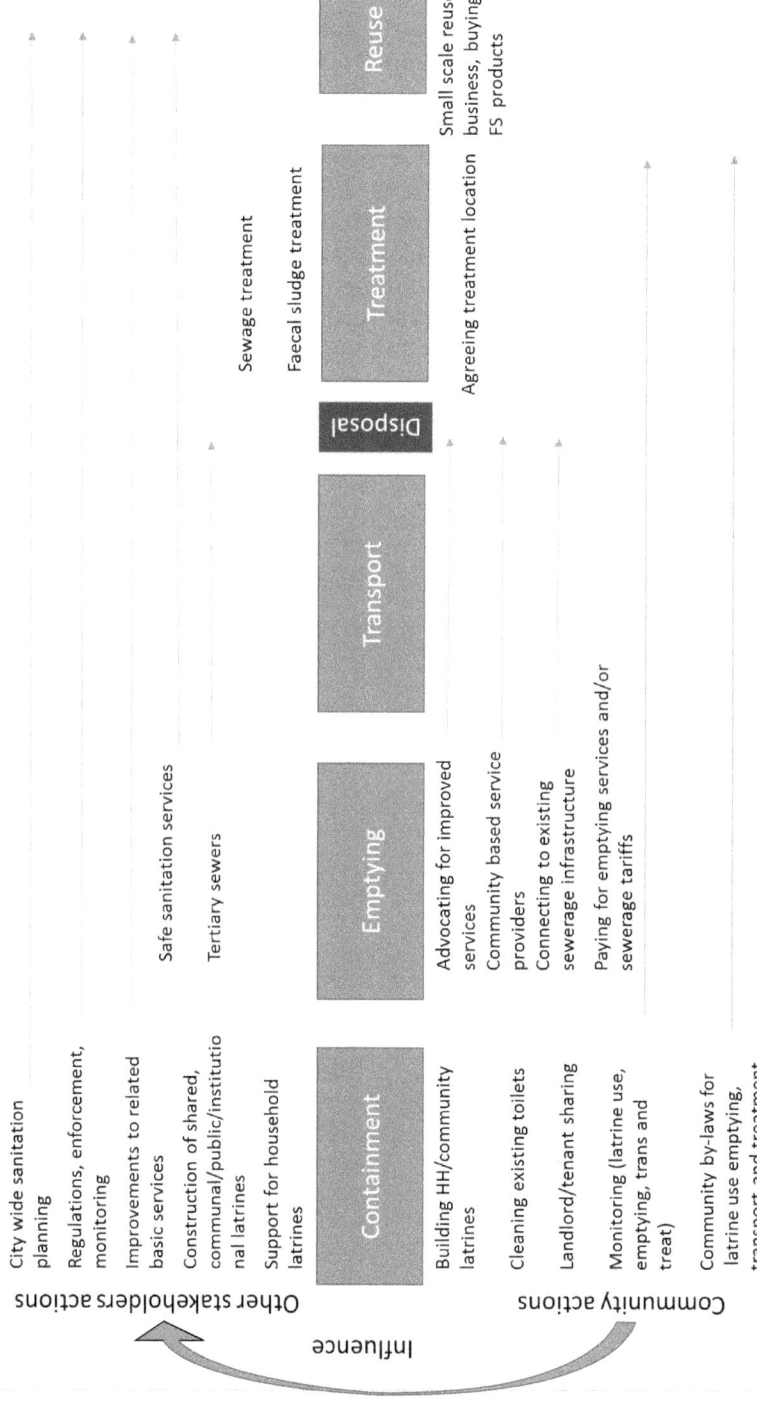

Figure 4.1 Actions along the sanitation chain

Revising and enforcing regulations across the sanitation chain

If used appropriately, local and national regulations can facilitate the actions that communities want to take to improve the supply of improved sanitation. Regulations are needed across the sanitation chain and may relate to the quality of toilets or the types of toilets that are allowed, designs for septic tanks, soak pits, and lined pits, and requirements for safe, hygienic FSM and treatment standards. In order for such regulations to be met, they need to be appropriate to the context: i.e. different standards may be required in slums to encourage first steps towards improved sanitation, as illustrated in the Nakuru example in Example 4.1. The regulations need to be well communicated, and training may be required to ensure that there is capacity within households, or among local construction workers, to comply with them.

For regulations to be effective, they need to be monitored and enforced in an appropriate manner. The challenge here may extend from a total lack of enforcement to inappropriately strict enforcement with unaffordable fines. The concept of 'smart enforcement' is used to describe a more purposeful

---

Example 4.1 – enforcing and revising regulation

In Choma, southern Zambia, a UNICEF Joint Monitoring Programme Team for sanitation coupled CLTS activities in peri-urban and urban areas with a legal enforcement approach. This established a mechanism for the enforcement of the Zambian Public Health Act, helping to ensure adequate sanitation in institutions, public places, and tenant households. As well as working with communities, the team worked with a diverse range of stakeholders, including town councils, chiefs, the judiciary, and the police, to create a legal enforcement team that complemented the community-based sanitation action groups. A fast-track court issued warnings. Landlords agreed on a date by which they had to build toilets for their tenants, otherwise they would receive a fine.

Source: Case Study 1: Choma, Zambia.

In Nakuru, Kenya, high standards of latrine construction enforced by the public health and planning departments were unattainable by poorer landlords and other urban residents. Therefore, Practical Action facilitated a participatory technology design process to achieve six latrine designs that were acceptable to community members, affordable to landlords, and met minimum standards for public health. Small wooden models of each were built and taken to communities to help people select a model they liked. Participants in this process included tenants, landlords, and their own qualified engineering staff. Public health representatives from the planning department were also engaged so that they understood the need to accept lower construction standards in this slum context.

Source: Case Study 12: Nakuru, Kenya; Pasteur and Prabhakaran, 2015.

design of regulations and enforcement approaches that embraces a range of measures that move beyond top-down penalty mechanisms (ISF-UTS and SNV, 2017). Enforcement can be more effective when there is collaboration between different stakeholders (e.g. local government and community volunteers), when different enforcement styles are considered (i.e. not simply financial penalties), and when the level of regulatory effort is appropriate to the risk that non-compliance poses to health or the environment (ISF-UTS and SNV, 2017).

Actions here are likely to involve working alongside local government to establish appropriate standards, regulations, and means of enforcement. Further action could involve working collaboratively to communicate the required standards, building capacity for implementation, and working together around monitoring and enforcement.

Safe capture and containment

The priorities for safe capture and containment will vary according to the situation and will be guided by the context. They include actions that can be taken directly by communities, perhaps with immediate effect, as well as actions that will require the engagement of external actors.

Actions that can be taken by communities

Some actions can be taken by communities themselves without requiring engagement with sanitation markets or incurring particularly significant costs. The scope of these actions will vary according to context, with denser urban slums and those with a high proportion of tenants being a little more limited in what is possible. However, in almost all cases, some actions are possible and can deliver a sense of progress while other negotiations are on-going. They can also act as an inspiration and a demonstration to other actors that the community is playing its part and is committed.

Actions can include the following:

- *Community commitment to ceasing OD*. Where this is feasible, such a public commitment should be a direct outcome of the community triggering process. This should include commitment to dispose safely of flying toilets and all faeces from babies and children.
- *Community monitoring of OD and unsafe FSM practices*. Community monitoring can be effective in encouraging behaviour change, particularly where there are consequences for failure to comply – for example, small fines are imposed or people/service providers are reported to the municipal authority for further action.
- *Construction of new latrines*. In places where this is feasible, this may be a relevant and possible action to immediately reduce unsafe defecation practices, even if latrines need to be upgraded or rebuilt later to meet urban standards.

- *Improvements to cleanliness and maintenance of existing toilet facilities.* This includes shared, communal, and public facilities, and aims to incentivize their use. This could involve renovations, repairs, emptying pits, limiting or controlling who uses them with a key or keys, employing a caretaker, regular cleaning, etc. This could contribute to eliminating OD and fixed-point OD. Agreeing maintenance rotas and incentives to maintain them will be important for shared facilities. It will also be important to ensure that these facilities are safe for all – for example, women at night.
- *Paying for safe FSM services.* This can include paying for services where they already exist. In places where networked sewerage exists, is functioning, and is affordable, this can involve connecting to these systems. The IUWASH programme in Indonesia was focused on triggering communities to connect unimproved and improved sanitation facilities to existing sewerage infrastructure, making them safely managed toilets (see Case Study 8). The ability to take these actions will be based on the price and affordability of these services – something usually beyond a community's control – as well as the availability of these services.
- *Community clean-ups of OD hotspots and common dumping grounds.* Alongside cleaning up, actions should be taken to deter people from continuing to use OD hotspots. In Nakuru, Kenya, people cut the grass in these areas to deter people from using them.

Example 4.2– Community actions

In peri-urban Gulariya, Nepal, households generally had secure tenure and sufficient space to construct a toilet. Many households, as in rural areas, were able to pay to construct or rehabilitate their own toilets and did not require additional support in terms of technical advice. There was an increased demand for slabs, which meant that local hardware dealers needed to source more of these to meet demand.

Source: Case Study 4: Gulariya, Nepal; Pasteur et al., 2016.

In Nakuru, Kenya, latrines were shared among renting households within a compound. These toilets were often in a very poor condition with shit all over the slab, sometimes overflowing, or with a superstructure that was falling down and no longer private. Residents initially took steps to clean up these latrines so that they could use them, until landlords took action to empty, rebuild, or renovate.

Source: Case Study 12: Nakuru, Kenya; Pasteur and Prabhakaran, 2015.

In Delhi, Nirmal Nari Awaas Samiti, a women's group, worked to renovate three existing community toilets, two of which were defunct and a third that was only partially functioning.

Source: Plan India, 2014.

> In Eritrea, a U-CLTS project run by UNICEF led to communities building substructures that were shared between households connected to indivudal superstructures.
>
> Source: Case Study 6: Himbirti, Eritrea.
>
> In Mathare 10, Nairobi, Kenya, a community organization for OD eradication was formed, there was an increase in toilet construction, community members demolished hanging toilets, and areas full of rubbish were cleaned.
>
> Source: Case Study 11: Mathare 10, Nairobi, Kenya.

Actions that require engagement with external stakeholders

Priorities for action on urban sanitation will be increasing the number of toilets available and improving the quality of existing toilets so that they are more accessible to all (including the elderly, people with disabilities, pregnant women, young children, etc.). There are a number of reasons why urban households are often less able to construct a safe toilet on their own:

- There is no space to build a toilet because the house takes up the entire plot.
- The family is renting and does not own the land or the house and therefore does not have permission to build a latrine.
- The household cannot afford the costs of latrine building and there is a lack of local building materials available.
- The house is owned but illegal from a planning perspective – i.e. it should not be there.
- The area has high ground water, is frequently flooded, or is built on rock or on stilts over a body of water – i.e. in a challenging environment.
- Toilets may need to meet legal standards for the safety and accessibility of the superstructure and substructure (e.g. lined pits or septic tanks), adding to the cost and complexity of construction.
- Limits are sometimes set regarding the number of people sharing a single facility, requiring additional facilities to be constructed.
- Construction may require help from an artisan and interaction with markets to buy hardware components, adding to the costs and complexity for the household or landlord.
- Markets for sanitation construction workers or necessary hardware supplies may not exist or may not be competitive or affordable.
- Households or landlords are often not able to raise the necessary finance for sanitation construction that meets the required standards.

The type of actions that can be supported by external actors to help resolve these issues include:

- participatory technology selection and design;
- participatory analysis of market systems and supply chains for toilet construction and hardware;
- capacity building for small and medium enterprises for component manufacture and sales, latrine building, faecal sludge service provision, container-based operators, etc.;
- improved access to finance and mobilizing savings;
- support for the building and good management of appropriately designed public and institutional toilets; and
- the use of container-based systems: for example, Clean Team (see Chapter 4 section 'Safe treatment, disposal and possible reuse'), Sanergy, Sanivation, etc. See https://www.cleanteamtoilets.com/, http://www.saner.gy/, and http://www.sanivation.com/. These systems are not yet at scale but their use looks promising for tenants and where conventional pit latrines cannot be built.

A range of existing tools and experiences provides guidance and ideas about how to boost the market for sanitation facilities. Applying the principles of a U-CLTS approach changes our perspective on some of these tools.

Participatory technology selection and design
Ensuring community engagement in the selection and design of sanitation options is a key part of improving sanitation in urban areas, where minimum levels of quality are more important than in rural settings. An interactive version of the *Compendium of Sanitation Systems and Technologies* has been developed (also available in French, Spanish, Vietnamese, and Nepalese) and is a useful starting point (Tilley et al., 2014). The *Community-Led Urban Environmental Sanitation Planning* manual (Lüthi et al., 2011) includes links to PowerPoint slides to introduce the compendium to stakeholders, and a suggested procedure for pre-selecting a set of technology options that would be suitable in a given context.

Building on the principles of a U-CLTS approach means using guides such as the compendium as a starting point, while allowing for innovation and flexibility in designs and technology choices. In choosing appropriate sanitation designs, questions of equity and social inclusion will be very important. Following the principles may lead us to think of a range of options at different price points and levels of sophistication that may help meet needs across households. A combination of community sanitation blocks (pay per use) and various household models may be needed – as will making sanitation inclusive for those who are disadvantaged or vulnerable.

TOOL 4.1 – Participatory technology development

What is it?	Participatory technology development (PTD) offers a methodology for ensuring that users participate in creating and selecting sanitation technologies that are appropriate and affordable for them. It provides an opportunity for users to express their traditional and often hidden knowledge and skills in partnership with designers and researchers.
Why use it?	Demand-led approaches to sanitation (including U-CLTS and sanitation marketing) encourage the participation of users to create, identify, and select appropriate sanitation technologies. Participatory design offers an established methodology to embrace the knowledge and skills of local users and suppliers of sanitation.
How to use it	It is important to convene a meeting of stakeholders, making sure to include end users. Participatory design sessions involve four stages: • *Stage 1*. Initial exploration of work – draw and label the existing sanitation technologies in their communities. • *Stage 2*. Discovery processes – each team identifies numerous potential design options. • *Stage 3*. Prototyping – create small- and medium-sized prototypes and estimate the material and labour costs of their prototypes. • *Stage 4*. Feedback – review the prototypes and provide feedback. The involvement of relevant municipal governments can help gain buy-in and ensure that plans meet the official minimum standards for public health.
Further guidance/ related case studies	Case Study 12: Nakuru, Kenya. Cole, 2013, http://www.communityledtotalsanitation.org/sites/communityledtotalsanitation.org/files/media/Frontiers_of_CLTS_Issue1_PartDesign_0.pdf

TOOL 4.2 – Participatory tools for socially inclusive design

What is it?	A number of practical tools have been developed to raise community awareness of the problems some users face in accessing and using latrines. They can be used to support the community to identify problems and possible solutions to improve the accessibility of latrines and to encourage vulnerable groups and individuals to participate actively by voicing their problems and opinions and contributing to problem-solving.

Why use it?	It raises community awareness about the barriers some members face, helps in the generation of community solutions, and gives a voice to those from vulnerable groups.
How to use it	Activities could include: • *Barrier analysis and solution tool.* A group exercise involving vulnerable and marginalized people or those in special circumstances, such as people with disabilities. It can also include Natural Leaders, local government health workers, those with vulnerable family members, and neighbours. Together they discuss the barriers and potential solutions to latrine use – these should include barriers related to safety. The end result should be the development of an action plan. Part of this could include a role-playing scenario and squatting activities (challenging people to squat when blindfolded, pregnant, injured, etc.). • *Accessibility and safety audits.* Facilitators evaluate the accessibility and safety of sanitation and associated facilities, identifying changes and improvements. These should be conducted by a mix of people, including disabled people, older people, women, etc. In relation to public latrines it can help analyse existing facilities to check their accessibility and also reduce vulnerabilities to violence through the consideration of users' safety. Partnerships between WASH and those working with vulnerable people, such as disability-sector organizations and institutions, can help strengthen these tools.
When would you use it?	These tools could be used in the assessment and preparation phase as well as during follow-up.
Further guidance	WEDC, 2017, https://wedc-knowledge.lboro.ac.uk/collections/equity-inclusion/general.html
	Jones, 2015, http://wedc.lboro.ac.uk/resources/learning/EI_Dialogue_circle_on_social_inclusion_guidance_note.pdf
	Wilbur and Jones, 2014, http://www.communityledtotalsanitation.org/sites/communityledtotalsanitation.org/files/Frontiers_of_CLTS_Issue3_Disabilities.pdf

Participatory analysis of market systems for toilet construction and hardware
One of the principles of a U-CLTS approach is to ensure replicability (avoiding hardware subsidies – if appropriate and possible), which puts a focus on improving the functioning of toilet construction markets. Part of this market system analysis needs to consider market segmentation, thinking about how to reach everyone, including those who may be the last to adopt new technologies.

Tools for participatory workshops are used to map the market system, identify the key actors and regulatory and policy issues, and identify why barriers exist. There is a guide to Participatory Market System Development online that shows how jointly developing a market map with all the key stakeholders can help identify the key barriers and issues that need to be overcome – and, crucially, improve relationships and trust between market actors. Part of the purpose is to empower actors lower down the value chain to expand their businesses (Tool 4.2).

Example 4.3 – Assessing market barriers

PSI has used market landscaping, firstly, to describe the total market systems, and secondly to identify market barriers. Used in West Africa, it involved in-depth interviews and focus group discussions with end users, landlords, value chain actors, and other key informants. The mapping exercise highlighted why markets were not working for the poor; these barriers were then identified and prioritized using a traffic light system.

Source: McHugh et al., 2015.

TOOL 4.3 – Participatory analysis of market systems for sanitation

What is it?	Participatory Market System Development (PMSD) makes markets more inclusive, reduces poverty on a large scale, and protects the environment. The approach, which has been developed over 12 years of fieldwork, is based on three broad principles: systems thinking, participation, and facilitation.
Why use it?	To harness the skills of all market chain actors, and to improve the relationships between different stakeholders. It enables a joint understanding of the market and suggestions for actions.
How to use it	The PMSD process works to build trust and a joint vision of change between these market actors, and helps them collectively identify obstacles and opportunities affecting their market system. The PMSD process starts with field staff analysing factors such as the potential to reach those most in need and a particular market's potential for growth. The next step is to get a better understanding of that market system, and the problems within it, by mapping out how the system fits together and researching each connection and market actor in detail.
	Facilitators then work to engage the key public and private actors within that market who can drive change – i.e. actually make the system work better. At the same time, the facilitators work to empower representatives of the marginalized actors (by improving

86 INNOVATIONS FOR URBAN SANITATION

their business language and helping them to better understand the market), putting them on a more capable and even footing to have an influence on how the process of change will take place. Staff facilitate the market actors in understanding where the opportunities and blockages are within the market system.

When would you use it?	As a follow-up activity to assess different options.
Further guidance	Participatory Market System Development, Practical Action, n.d.a, http://www.pmsdroadmap.org/

TOOL 4.4 – Supply chain analysis

What is it?	Supply chain analysis is a diagnostic of the sanitation supply chain. It focuses on commonly found or preferred products and services for improved sanitation. It includes interviews with supply chain actors, including construction material suppliers, producers of prefabricated concrete products, and masons, as well as local finance organizations and service providers.
Why use it?	Different locations have different supply chains, with different sources of products and services. The supply chain for sanitation includes not only materials such as latrine pans, cement, steel, and zinc sheets but safe emptying, transportation, and treatment of sewerage. Many construction material suppliers act as importers, wholesalers, and retailers. Latrines are a slow-moving consumer durable (i.e. low frequency, lumpy sales), thus margins for latrine products and services are often tighter for masons than other activities.
	Supply chains for sanitation may be fragmented – i.e. households have to collect materials rather than buy a single-priced final latrine product. Supply chain analysis can help understand the transaction costs for households, who may have to visit at least two actors to collect the necessary materials. Supply chain analysis might also be used for the marketing of products and services.
How to use it	It is used to analyse the materials and products for latrine construction: cement, iron bars (rebar), wire mesh, and PVC pipes, as well as certain prefabricated sanitation products (pans, pipes, cleansing materials, pipe fittings).
	It can help in assessing labour availability and access to credit, and in understanding the supply chain actors such as wholesalers

	and retailers. It is also important to understand where supply chain actors mostly get their customers, i.e. through personal contacts.
When would you use it?	In the assessment and preparation stage, to understand the availability of wholesalers and retailers as well as supplies in market areas such as district headquarters and business hubs and the availability of masons employed to construct latrines. It is also important to understand the need for finance – i.e. whether wholesalers, retailers, masons, or ring producers need loans to run their business.
Further guidance	IUWASH, 2015, https://www.iuwashplus.or.id/cms/wp-content/uploads/2017/04/Guide-to-Urban-Sanitation-Promotion-EN.pdf

Capacity building for small and medium enterprises and informal actors
Those who lack basic services are likely to depend on small- to medium-scale businesses and informal service providers. These enterprises and informal sector actors are likely to emerge in the participatory market systems analysis above. Water and Sanitation for the Urban Poor stresses the need to 'support entrepreneurs with capacity development and start-up finance. Equally... [there is a need to work] with institutions to (a) improve the regulatory framework and provide the entrepreneurs with clear guidelines for complying with local laws; and (b) update policies and strategies to reflect the reality in any given location' (WSUP, 2014: 52). Capacity development might include training artisans in new latrine designs. It might also involve offering wider technical, management, and financial support to encourage existing enterprises to expand their businesses, and for others to extend their business areas to include work on sanitation.

Improved access to finance and mobilizing savings
A range of financing options could be made available to help communities afford and spread the costs of investing in improved sanitation:

- involvement from local businesses in donating materials or providing funding;
- revolving funds to purchase hardware;
- use of savings;
- payment by instalments;
- microcredit products through banks or microfinance institutions; and
- supporting community sanitation blocks by adding value to the waste by selling biogas or compost.

Examples are given in Example 4.4 overleaf.

Example 4.4 – Improving access to finance

In Kenya, Umande Trust has built bio-centres in low-income communities in Nairobi, Nakuru, and elsewhere. These are public toilets that generate biogas from faecal waste. The bio-centres are managed by community groups that earn income from charging for access to the toilets, enabling them to pay wages and maintenance costs. The biogas feeds a kitchen that can be hired out for cooking.

Source: Case Study 12: Nakuru, Kenya; Pasteur and Prabhakaran, 2015.

In Blantyre, Malawi, Slum Dweller Federation members have accessed a range of sources of finance to improve their sanitation situation. However, having their own finance accumulated through the daily savings of members has allowed them to make their own investments. By 2014, daily savings had enabled the construction of almost 700 eco-sanitation toilets, shared by an average of three families each.

Source: Mitlin, 2014.

In Indonesia, the price of healthy toilets ranges between Rp 650,000 and Rp 2,500,000 (approximately £35 to £130) and the community can buy them using a microfinance scheme with a certain amount of upfront costs and weekly instalments of as little as Rp 10,000 to Rp 15,000.

Source: IUWASH, 2015.

In 2012, WASTE initially partnered with the Zambian National Building Society; however, the loan application criteria were too strict and the process too lengthy – applications had to be sent to Lusaka to be signed off. In 2015, WASTE partnered with the Community Empowerment Fund, a local microfinance institution. With their head office in Kabwe, they are closer to the ground and the process is faster. In addition, they spent time designing an appropriate loan. To apply for a loan, a bill of quantity is filled out that states the different materials needed to build a urine-diverting dry toilet; households tick boxes corresponding to the materials they need. This means that loans can be reduced if households are able to provide the materials themselves.

Source: Case Study 9: Kabwe, Zambia; Myers, 2016.

The Centre for Community Organisation and Development has supported communities in accessing improved sanitation and water through a revolving fund called Mchenga. This fund is the only finance instrument in Malawi that provides water and sanitation loans.

Source: CCODE, 2014.

Support for public and institutional toilets
Public toilets are in public places and are used by people when they are away from home, for example at transport and commercial hubs. They differ from communal toilets, which are shared by a set number of households and are primarily for domestic use. Occasionally, when a community lives near a public place, the two can be combined. The distinction is important when it comes to building, operation, management, and FSM services, as there is often less community ownership for public toilets (WSUP, 2016). However, where outside assistance will be necessary, with the right incentives community groups could potentially take charge of their management.

Any urban sanitation intervention should also consider an institutional sanitation component. Safely managed sanitation will be needed at institutions such as hospitals and schools.

> **Example 4.5 – Community-managed facilities**
>
> In Hawassa, Ethiopia, a recently constructed and pay-to-use toilet and shower block is being managed by a Natural Leaders' group.
>
> *Source*: Case Study 5: Hawassa, Ethiopia.
>
> In Nakuru, Kenya, as part of the U-CLTS project, the Umande Trust built a public toilet in the middle of a market. It is also a biogas generator with a combined kitchen and meeting space that can be hired out. The Trust has signed a memorandum of understanding with a youth organization that will take over responsibility for running and managing the facility.
>
> *Source*: Case Study 12: Nakuru, Kenya; Pasteur and Prabhakaran, 2015.

Tip 4.1 – Right to sanitation and vulnerable groups

Think about the right to sanitation of vulnerable groups such as street dwellers or homeless people who rely on public places for urination and defecation. What alternatives are there for this community to practise adequate, safe, and dignified sanitation?

Joshi and Morgan (2007) reported on the sanitation practices of pavement dwellers:

- Young boys often defecate, urinate, and even bathe in the open.
- Defecating, urinating, or even bathing on the streets are not preferred options for adolescent males.
- Young adolescent girls report that 'public toilets are not safe places to visit'.

Men can choose to bathe, defecate, and urinate in public; women experience much greater discomfort and risk in doing so, given the conditioning that this behaviour is not socially acceptable.

Safe emptying and transportation

In urban areas, achieving a shit-free environment will almost always entail engaging with systems for safer emptying, transportation, and treatment of faecal sludge from on-site sanitation systems. The key issues and priorities will be identified in the situation analysis. Faecal waste or shit flow diagrams are a particularly useful tool here to highlight the key areas for action (see Chapter 3 section 'Institutional advocacy tools and tactics').

Using a U-CLTS approach does not necessarily mean expecting communities to play the leading role in delivering safe emptying and transportation systems. These are likely to require collaboration with external systems to a greater or lesser extent. However, the principles of U-CLTS would influence the strategy by ensuring a focus on the following:

- *Participation and empowerment.* People will be mobilized to advocate for improved emptying and transportation services by the service providers.
- *Demand creation resulting from triggering.* The focus on behaviour change should generate demand for pit-emptying services and reduce the prevalence of unsafe practices.
- *Total sanitation.* Everyone in a given area needs to be able to access safe FSM and sewerage services when needed and a focus should be maintained on creating viable businesses.

Actions that can be taken by communities

The scope for communities to take their own action will depend on the context: for example, land availability and ownership for constructing toilets, connection to sewers, pit-emptying services, etc. However, whatever the starting point, it is important to find some opportunity for making a difference within the community that is meaningful and can be the starting point for greater engagement with external actors.

Actions could include:

- establishing agreed cleaning, maintenance, and emptying regimes for shared toilets;
- alerting landlords and other authorities who might have responsibility for emptying toilets when they are full;
- ensuring commitment from toilet owners to stop harmful practices such as the emptying of pits or septic tanks in the open or into open drains when they are full – instead they should engage a pit-emptying service that will dispose of the waste at a designated facility;
- ensuring commitment to appropriate hygienic disposal of infant faeces and diapers;
- establishing a safe and hygienic community-based or community-managed pit-emptying service (although this will also require integration with external actors);

- being vigilant that no FSM service providers are dumping faecal waste within the community – or anywhere outside it, except in a designated treatment facility; and
- articulating demands for improved emptying services by external actors by campaigning or communicating with relevant external actors – this includes lobbying local government for affordable and hygienic FSM services if they do not exist.

> **Example 4.6 – Community involvement in FSM**
>
> The community of Nala in Nepal has around 400 households. Following the participatory CLUES methodology, the community opted for simplified sewers, together with a small local treatment plant using an anaerobic baffle reactor and a horizontal-flow, gravel-bed filter. A users' committee is responsible for the long-term operation and maintenance of the system.
>
> *Source:* Lüthi et al., 2011; Myers et al., 2016.

Actions that require engagement with external actors

As noted above, there is a high likelihood that action to address safe emptying and transportation will require engagement with actors beyond the community. These actors might include the municipal authority, private providers, urban planners, public health officials, and other NGOs, each of whom might have a different role to play in addressing the issues at stake.

Building the capacity of informal pit emptiers
Informal pit emptiers are key stakeholders who:

- know their customers;
- may provide a flexible and cost-effective service; and
- are able to access more challenging locations with their smaller-scale operating equipment.

However, they often face discrimination and social exclusion as a result of their unpleasant work, which is often a last resort and highly risky to their and their customers' health. Because manual pit emptying is often discouraged by municipalities and because of the disruption and smells caused, they often work under the cover of darkness and sometimes with the help of drugs or drink as a coping mechanism. The simplistic action of outlawing them does not make their services more hygienic or provide alternative services. It is important to ensure that the voices and concerns of informal pit emptiers are heard. They should not be forced to take business risks that could push them further into poverty. Clean uniforms and protective and improved emptying equipment help raise the status and attractiveness of informal pit emptiers

> **Example 4.7 – Capacity development for FSM**
>
> In Bangladesh, Practical Action has supported two groups of informal pit emptiers to form co-operatives providing mechanical desludging services, and to enter into service agreements with the municipality. They are able to lease pumping equipment from the municipality, and they can now operate freely during the daytime, charge more predictable rates to customers, and dispose of the waste safely.
>
> *Source*: Stevens et al., 2015, 2017.
>
> In Gulariya, Nepal, Practical Action has worked alongside the municipality to support the provision of a sludge removal service that is appropriate to the needs of small peri-urban householders. Furthermore, the sludge will be composted, providing a more ecologically sustainable solution to the sludge management problem. The enterprise is a public–private partnership and employs local people.
>
> *Source*: Case Study 4: Gulariya, Nepal; Pasteur and Prabhakaran, 2015.

(Blackett and Hawkins, 2017). In several countries, there have been efforts to make their services more hygienic with the use of simple equipment such as buckets, scoops, or gulpers, and to encourage the wearing of protective clothing. This has helped to improve their image and their social acceptance.

There is extensive scope for technical training of pit emptiers to enhance the health and safety of the service, the workers, and the wider public. Appropriate technologies have been developed to reach pits that large tankers are unable to access. These may need to be introduced, adapted, or improved in collaboration with the pit emptiers to ensure that they are affordable, effective, and sustainable. To ensure safe disposal of sludge after pits have been emptied, there is a need for engagement with formal service providers (the utility company or the municipality) so that informal pit emptiers are able to access appropriate treatment facilities. It may require considerable effort to convince utilities or the municipality that informal service providers can operate in a safe and effective manner, but a number of examples exist where a successful outcome has been achieved. Formalization or registration of pit-emptier groups and the establishment of agreed contracts for operation are typically required and have been usefully employed in Faridpur, Bangladesh (Stevens et al., 2015).

Safe treatment, disposal, and possible reuse

The final step of the sanitation chain is the safe treatment, disposal, and possible reuse of faecal sludge. It is important to note that treatment can be missed and disposal can occur directly after collection and/or transportation: for example, burying pit latrines.

It will be important to ensure that shit is not entering other residential areas. There are limited things communities will be able to do. However, as in safe emptying and transportation, U-CLTS principles can still influence practice by focusing on the following:

- *Participation and empowerment.* Communities co-operating in decision-making processes around the location of treatment plants or the services they are offered.
- *Demand creation resulting from triggering.* Mobilizing communities to take action if unsafe effluent is being disposed of locally: i.e. shit is entering their communities from outside.
- *Total sanitation*: Ensuring that affordable services are available that do not lead to shit re-entering the community or polluting other areas.

> **Example 4.8 – Container-based sanitation**
>
> A promising option for scalable, inclusive, and safe FSM services where other low-cost options are not feasible is container-based sanitation (CBS). It has the potential to be used by tenants and in challenging environments, as no permanent infrastructure is needed. CBS is based on a business model linked to individual toilets that collect excreta in a sealable cartridge that can then be removed and replaced with an empty one. It has been described as a low-cost way to provide safe collection, transportation, and treatment.
>
> An example of this is The Clean Team, a social enterprise based in Kumasi, Ghana that provides safe and affordable toilets for families. They charge a weekly fee with no upfront payment. Containers are picked up weekly from households who are then given empty ones. The waste is the safely disposed of at Kumasi sewage works.
>
> CBS services are still in the early stages of development, and their sustainability and affordability at scale is being tested. In addition to the examples above, their potential is being explored by different organizations using different business models in Kenya, Madagascar, Haiti, and Peru.
>
> *Source*: EY and WSUP, 2017.

Associated waste streams

In many cases, triggering can lead to a significant motivation to address solid waste and drainage issues within the community alongside human excreta challenges. Often these are seen as related issues as solid and liquid waste both create an unpleasant living environment and are carriers of disease. Due to a lack of appropriate services and a lack of enforced regulation, people often use pit latrines for the disposal of solid waste such as sanitary towels (menstrual hygiene waste) or children's nappies, as well as general household waste, including dangerous items such as razor blades and knives, and bulky items

94 INNOVATIONS FOR URBAN SANITATION

such as tins or plastic. The presence of such refuse in the pits makes them fill up faster and makes them more difficult to empty. Gulpers or other suction-based pit or tank emptiers do not work well when there is a large amount of solid waste in the faecal sludge, and the removal of solid waste that has been mixed with faecal sludge is inevitably unhygienic.

Stagnant waste water from household washing is a critical health hazard in many countries, particularly increasing the risk of malaria. Simple actions can be taken to improve drainage.

Actions that can be taken by communities

Examples of actions that can be taken directly by communities include:

- community campaigns to clear areas where solid waste has accumulated – this might also include cutting grass and general tidying to help encourage the maintenance of clean households and the wider environment;
- construction of household soakaways, drainage channels, and washing platforms to eliminate stagnant water around the household;
- clearing of drainage systems, including storm drains, to eliminate stagnant water and reduce flood risk within the community;
- community plans to reduce solid waste in latrines – for example, SatoPans (http://www.sato.lixil.com/) can introduce a water seal, make it harder to add waste, and are increasingly available at low cost;
- establishing plans for waste management, collection, recycling, etc. if they do not already exist – these can be proposed to local authorities or community groups for implementation;
- establishing a waste collection or recycling business, although this is likely to require collaboration with external actors;
- promoting a range of options for managing menstrual hygiene products; and
- establishing sanctions for the dumping of waste in the community.

TOOL 4.5 – Solid waste calculations

What is it?	Calculating the amount of solid waste produced can help illustrate the magnitude of the sanitation problem.
Why use it?	The calculations of quantities of solid waste produced by the community should lead to further questions and discussions: for example, where does all the solid waste go? What are the possible effects of having so much solid waste on the ground? These types of questions will get the community starting to think for themselves about the possible impacts.

How to use it	Households are asked to calculate how much rubbish they produce. The households' waste figures can then be added up to produce a total for the whole community. A daily figure can be multiplied to know how much solid waste is produced per week, per month, or per year. The quantities can add up to a matter of tonnes, which may surprise the community.
When would you use it?	During a triggering session or as a post-triggering follow-up activity.
Related case studies	Case Study 5: Hawassa, Ethiopia.

> **Example 4.9 – Waste collection and income generation**
>
> Waste collection is an income-generating opportunity that can transform U-CLTS Natural Leaders into waste and sanitation entrepreneurs. In Hawassa, Ethiopia, Plan Ethiopia built the capacity of Natural Leaders to establish a waste collection business. This meant that when they were regularly visiting compounds to collect waste they could also observe and discuss sanitation issues with the residents. Charging for waste removal gave them a small income which further facilitated their role as a sanitation Natural Leader. A key challenge they faced was accessing a site for the safe disposal of the waste they were collecting.
>
> *Source*: Case Study 5: Hawassa, Ethiopia; Myers et al., 2016; Myers, 2016.

Actions that require engagement with external actors

There will also be a need to engage with external actors to improve solid waste and waste water management. This can include:
- lobbying municipalities to allocate budget for improving drainage infrastructure in the settlement and across the wider city;
- lobbying for regular waste collection systems and/or emptying of skips or other secondary storage facilities;
- capacity building for community waste collection and recycling entrepreneurs who may require support with transport, storage/sorting space, and access to a place where they can dispose of non-recyclable waste; and
- the provision of waste collection services by municipalities or by public or private utility companies.

Dos and don'ts for integrating U-CLTS across the sanitation chain

Table 4.1 Dos and don'ts: integrating U-CLTS across the sanitation chain

Dos	Don'ts
1. Focus on empowerment and innovation, universal access, and collective behaviour change.	1. Focus only on the provision of toilets – ensure that systems are in place to address all relevant aspects of the sanitation chain.
2. Develop a collaborative strategy with inputs from communities and other relevant stakeholders.	2. Assume that actions to address sanitation cannot be taken by communities.
3. Draw on good practice in urban sanitation to design actions.	3. Assume that the community can deliver all actions required to strengthen the sanitation chain.
4. Involve all actors in the sanitation chain. Work closely with community leadership, Natural Leaders, and local entrepreneurs, as well as existing service providers, whether private, government, or parastatal.	4. Forget the need for finance and savings.
5. Start with 'small immediate doable actions'. Community motivation will be enhanced by short-term positive achievements.	5. Focus on hardware only. People and collective behaviour change are at the heart of achieving total urban sanitation.
6. Ensure widespread participation (community and other stakeholders) in the analysis of market systems or technology selection.	6. Think about sanitation in isolation from solid and liquid waste management.
7. Build the capacity of SMEs, e.g. for sanitation hardware supply, construction, pit emptying, solid waste collection, etc. This can improve the sustainability of services, strengthen the local economy, and provide more affordable services.	7. Ignore successful interventions from other approaches.
8. Identify and work with people who may be disadvantaged and need additional support or require adapted technologies.	
9. Think about the finance options to ensure that sanitation elements can be implemented: e.g. savings groups, low-cost loans, subsidies for materials, etc.	
10. Promote the enforcement of national regulations to ensure action to improve sanitation. However, where regulations are not relevant to low-income communities, lobby for them to be adapted.	

Notes for users

CHAPTER 5
Stage 4: Maintaining momentum

Abstract

U-CLTS is about the engagement and empowerment of communities, stakeholders, and institutions to achieve improved sanitation outcomes for all. This chapter looks at the necessary follow-up, monitoring, verification, and certification needed to harness this enthusiasm and ensure that planned actions and behaviour changes take place and are sustained over time. It is important that behaviours are maintained and planned actions go ahead. It suggests achievable goals that could be set and rightly celebrated on the journey towards total sanitation.

Keywords: Follow-up; monitoring; verification and certification; sustainability; sanitation goals; Natural Leaders.

Key messages

- Building capacity and supporting Natural Leaders and CBOs to maintain and monitor progress in an inclusive and participatory manner will aid sustainability.
- It is important to establish clear and attainable sanitation goals that can be monitored and verified for certification and celebration. Over time, these may be adopted by authorities.
- Once sanitation outcomes have been achieved, impact can be enhanced by continuing to encourage Natural Leaders and emerging champions to organize and expand their sphere of influence for change.

Purpose of maintaining momentum

Maintaining momentum is about ensuring that planned actions and behaviour changes take place and are sustained over time to achieve the desired sanitation goals and outcomes. Initial goals could be based around safe containment of faecal sludge before moving towards the more complex challenges further down the sanitation service chain. This may also involve moving beyond sanitation alone, to address wider water and hygiene issues, solid waste management, drainage, or other community concerns.

http://dx.doi.org/10.3362/9781780447360.005

A U-CLTS approach should empower local people – as individuals or within community organizations – to maintain the momentum of change. This could involve:

- encouraging the building or maintenance of household or compound sanitation provision;
- engaging or lobbying landlords, service providers, market actors, and others to ensure that they deliver sanitation services or hardware to which they have committed;
- formal monitoring of progress towards sanitation goals agreed by the community in the action plan;
- verifying and celebrating sanitation achievements over time;
- monitoring sustainability of behaviour change and other achievements; and
- moving beyond sanitation to tackle a wider range of issues.

Ensuring that these processes are driven by the community and that they are working towards total coverage of the defined community or neighbourhood is key to the U-CLTS approach.

There are four elements to the process of maintaining momentum:

1. *Follow-up.* Regular encouragement along with formal tracking of progress can ensure that the process does not lose momentum and fail. People tend to quickly forget the disgust and anger that motivated them during triggering, so action must be facilitated while that determination to change is still strong. Due to the complexity of addressing urban sanitation issues, the need for regular follow-up visits is particularly important to help people maintain their direction or drive for change.
2. *Monitoring.* Monitoring should be undertaken alongside regular follow-up to assess and measure progress more formally. This will help community members and external facilitators ensure that they are on track. Monitoring tools should be used in such a way as to motivate further action and continually improve sanitation standards.
3. *Verification, certification, and celebration.* Achieving a shit-free environment is far more complex in urban areas than ODF in rural settings due to the characteristics of the urban sanitation context outlined in the introduction (for example, defining the extent of one community, the different manifestations of faecal contamination from fixed point OD to flying toilets, unsafe emptying, etc. – see Table 1.2 and Figure 1.2). However, it is important to acknowledge even small steps of progress towards improved sanitation and to regularly celebrate successes. The behaviour changes that are verified, certified, and celebrated may vary from one urban context to another.
4. *Sustainability.* Once a community has achieved a measure of improved sanitation, it is important for the behaviour change to be sustained over the long term. Mechanisms need to be put in place to ensure long-term follow-up on sanitation, as well as motivating people to move beyond

basic elimination of unsafe sanitation practices towards achieving a wider range of water- and sanitation-related outcomes, including solid waste and waste water management.

Follow-up

There are complex challenges involved in addressing urban sanitation and conflicts can often arise. Therefore, regular encouragement, problem-solving, and conflict resolution may be needed to keep processes and activities moving within urban communities. Follow-up also involves checking the progress of service providers in fulfilling any commitments they have made, and holding them to account. There is also the need to maintain engagement with local actors and to be aware of broader urban plans that may affect the community.

Follow-up can be done by Natural Leaders, NGO staff, health visitors or community development officers, community groups, children, local leaders, or other relevant local actors. A wide range of tools and methods can be used, ranging from house-to-house visits and community meetings to exchanges and competitions. Many methods, such as visits or exchanges, are more feasible in a dense urban context. However, community meetings can be more challenging due to people's busy lives.

A key to successful follow-up is to engage a wide range of actors, working through a variety of channels with an overarching strategic plan. It is critical to start follow-up promptly after triggering and action planning to ensure that any momentum gained is not lost.

TACTIC 5.1 – Sanitation ambassadors

What is it?	Identify, encourage, and support high-profile ambassadors for improved sanitation.
Why use it?	Role models can help spread messages about the need for improved sanitation and hygiene and the need to maintain and build upon gains made.
How to use it	Engage and inspire high-profile local or national personalities to identify with, endorse, and support the sanitation campaign. At a local level, these could be influential and respected religious, spiritual, or political leaders or other local celebrities, who can persuade their followers to adopt hygienic behaviour.
	Similarly, at a national level, sports, television, radio, film, or political personalities can be engaged to make public statements through a range of media channels: for example, posters, TV adverts, speeches, radio jingles, etc.
When would you use it?	This can be used throughout the process.

TOOL 5.1 – Community exchange visits

What is it? Members of one community visit another community to review and encourage progress.

Why use it? Exchange visits can foster peer-to-peer support and learning. They can also encourage competition between communities and between local government areas. For the visitors, it shows what they are capable of achieving and they come away armed with new ideas and approaches. For the hosts, it can help Natural Leaders and volunteers feel appreciated and recognized for the work in which they are engaging. The hosts also have to explain their project to a new and interested audience, seeing their own projects afresh through new eyes.

How to use it The proximity of communities in urban areas provides a good opportunity for exchange visits. Community members can visit another similar community that has made progress on improving its sanitation situation. This activity may be a one-off or may happen regularly over the duration of a project. Effective facilitation is important to ensure that learning and reflection take place. Prior to the visit it is important that the community being visited is prepared and key informants are there to show the visitors around. It is important to build in time for visitors to reflect on what they have learned.

In Ethiopia, World Vision used exchange visits between communities to encourage and celebrate progress. Each community elected a seven-member sanitation task force. Periodically, exchange visits were organized between villages during which the seven members between them visited all the households and assessed the toilets using an agreed checklist. Finally, the task force would come together, compare the rankings, and celebrate those projects that were best.

Further guidance/ related case studies
Case Study 2: Eight towns in Ethiopia.
Case Study 8: IUWASH, Indonesia.
IUWASH, 2015, https://www.iuwashplus.or.id/cms/wp-content/uploads/2017/04/Guide-to-Urban-Sanitation-Promotion-EN.pdf
Myers et al., 2016, www.communityledtotalsanitation.org/sites/communityledtotalsanitation.org/files/The_Addis_Agreement_CLTS_urban_0.pdf

TACTIC 5.2 – Use of traditional and social media

What is it? Use of traditional media (newspaper, radio, TV, etc.) as well as social media (Facebook, twitter, blogs, etc.) to promote sanitation messages.

Why use it? The use of U-CLTS tools and tactics will need to be embedded into a wider behaviour change communication strategy. Both traditional and social media can be used to reinforce messages and ensure that all community members are reached.

How to use it Both traditional and social media can be used as part of a wider set of behaviour change communication tools. There is significant potential for accessing media and social media for follow-up in urban areas due to the range and accessibility of different media streams. Mainstream media (radio, TV, newspapers) can be used for promoting good sanitation practice.

Billboards can be used for communicating in markets, at road intersections, etc. to illustrate improved hygiene behaviours.

Film has also been used as a dissemination tool for sanitation messages. In Gulariya, Nepal, a short video documentary (4–5 minutes) outlining the oral faecal pathway was regularly used in initiating discussions around sanitation in communities. Furthermore, a much longer comedic film called *Charpi Bihe* (*Toilet Marriage*) was produced by national government for sanitation promotion purposes. Filmed in the Nepali language and set within the cultural background of the country, this comedy involves a lovestruck couple whose desire to marry is thwarted due to continued OD by the girl's father, until he is finally convinced to build a toilet. They finally marry and the ritual wedding dance is performed around the new toilet. The film was successful in connecting people to the issue of sanitation in an informal and entertaining way.

Facebook, blogs, WhatsApp and other social media can be used to spread messages, promote debate, and highlight good and bad practice through photo sharing. In Mathare 10, Kenya, blogs and WhatsApp have been used to promote messaging about local sanitation issues. Photographs of discarded rubbish, flying toilets, etc. would often be posted by people from neighbouring areas to bring the problems directly to the attention of local residents.

Further guidance/ related case studies	Case Study 4: Gulariya, Nepal.
	Case Study 11: Mathare 10, Nairobi, Kenya.
	Musyoki, 2010, http://www.communityledtotalsanitation.org/sites/communityledtotalsanitation.org/files/media/Mathare_blog_all.pdf

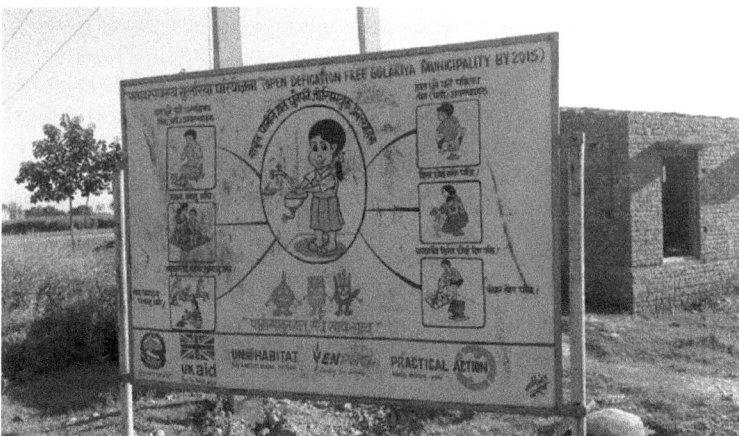

Figure 5.1 Billboard promoting handwashing at key times, Gulariya, Nepal
Source: Katherine Pasteur.

TACTIC 5.3 – Women's groups

What is it?	Women's groups, female savings and loans groups, mothers' groups, etc. are particularly effective in promoting the sustainability of health and sanitation interventions.
Why use it?	Where women are already organized for other purposes, they can easily be mobilized to support sanitation campaigns as the impact of sanitation is typically close to their heart.
How to use it	Women's groups can be invited to share their views on sanitation, hygiene, menstrual hygiene, and how poor sanitation has an impact on them and their families. Ask their advice and ideas on how best to encourage action within the community to improve sanitation, and help them to identify the roles they can play. One way may be to strengthen their capacity and potential for disseminating messages on sanitation and hygiene, whether through their existing regular meetings, special events, or door-to-door sanitation promotion visits.
Further guidance/ related case studies	Case Study 4: Gulariya, Nepal. Plan India, 2014, http://www.communityledtotalsanitation.org/sites/communityledtotalsanitation.org/files/media/UCLTS_Delhi_Report_Plan.pdf

Example 5.1 – Engaging women's groups

There are many different examples of engaging women's groups in sanitation behaviour change campaigns. A Plan India project in Delhi mobilized and trained women through a group called Nirmal Nari Awaas Samiti (NNAS). One of the first actions of the NNAS was to conduct mapping activities with the community. This helped them understand what resources were available and where, as well as the major gaps and challenges. The members then went on to conduct several health and sanitation workshops and carried out door-to-door campaigns to convince people about the necessity of toilets and water purity. Two NNAS leaders are now the key sanitation advocates for the community, often holding impromptu short training workshops on the street. They are known now as the 'go-to' people to find solutions to community problems.

Source: Plan India, 2014.

Monitoring

Progress monitoring is critical for keeping track of the status of community actions, behaviour change, and the actions of external stakeholders. Regular progress monitoring driven by facilitating agencies also helps ensure that progress is smooth, that bottlenecks are addressed promptly, and that learning is gathered to feed into future practice. Monitoring should extend beyond the immediate achievement of sanitation outcomes to ensure that they are sustained over time.

Monitoring may be facilitated by local community actors such as Natural Leaders, Community Health Volunteers, etc., and by external players such as NGO staff, public health staff, etc. Developing simple but effective methodologies and clearly allocating responsibilities are keys to success.

The types of indicators selected to monitor progress of U-CLTS are likely to be different to those used in rural CLTS. In rural areas, proxy indicators for achieving ODF include construction of household toilets, evidence of use, cleanliness of former OD sites, and evidence of handwashing facilities. In urban areas, indicators may include the above where relevant, but in addition it may be necessary to consider the following measures:

- improved cleanliness or maintenance of existing toilets;
- reductions in the number of people sharing toilets;
- improvements in the quality and standard of facilities (e.g. upgrading to lined pits or septic tanks, or improved superstructure);
- regular use of handwashing facilities;
- toilets that can be accessed by all sectors of the community (including disabled people, pregnant women, the elderly, children, homeless people, etc.);
- safe disposal of infant faeces, nappies, sanitary towels, etc.;
- availability, accessibility, and affordability of public and institutional toilets (e.g. in market places, bus stations, medical centres, municipal offices, etc.);
- adequate provision of safe sanitation facilities by landlords and enforcement where they are lacking;
- the performance of different institutions in terms of their roles and effectiveness in facilitating sanitation and waste disposal;
- regularity and affordability of emptying services for pits or septic tanks;
- regularity and affordability of solid waste collection services;
- enforcement of regulations and penalties relating to waste dumping or ineffective waste collection services; and
- monitoring of water quality to ensure that local legal standards are being met.

> **Example 5.2 – Community-based monitoring**
>
> In Fort Dauphin, Madagascar, community members agreed a set of criteria for rating toilets on maintenance, cleanliness, handwashing, availability of soap, etc. Each month a group of health volunteers would walk round the community and rank every latrine. Neighbours were also given the opportunity to rate each other's latrines over three months, with results presented on a whiteboard situated in a communal place. Those families who have maintained high standards over three months are presented with a small incentive in a presentation ceremony, which encourages positive behavioural change.
>
> *Source*: Case Study 3: Fort Dauphin, Madagascar; Myers et al., 2016; Azafady, 2015.
>
> Child Health Monitors is a children's group. Each group has five '*panchs*' or ministers who contribute to their neighbourhood's development. They are in charge of drains, water, cleanliness, toilets, and health respectively. CHM runs numerous awareness events in the community on sanitation, menstrual health, water issues, and hygiene. For eight months during CHM's 'Seeti Bajao' (whistleblowing) campaign, *panchs* would set out each morning to ensure that their neighbourhood stayed ODF. This activity is now run on a periodic basis.
>
> *Panchs* were also encouraged to use mobile phones to film rubbish piles, blocked drains, and other discrepancies in behaviour.
>
> *Source*: Plan India, 2014.

A wide range of tools for monitoring CLTS in rural areas can be transferred directly to the urban context. Many methods can be more effective in urban areas due to the density of population: for example, community exchanges are easier due to closer proximity. Additional tools are required for monitoring institutional responsibilities and performance along the sanitation chain, which can be used by the community to hold stakeholders to account. Examples of and experience with these types of tools are limited.

> **TOOL 5.2 – Visual monitoring**
>
> | | |
> |---|---|
> | What is it? | Using a visual map displayed in public to show progress towards total sanitation in a community. |
> | Why use it? | Making it public ensures that everyone is able to monitor progress. |
> | How to use it | This could be based on the community map created during triggering or action planning. Colours or symbols can be used to show: when areas of OD have been cleaned up; households or compounds with improved sanitation; locations of public toilets, etc. This includes creating a map of all households and public places and marking |

STAGE 4: MAINTAINING MOMENTUM   107

them once sanitation facilities are considered adequate. If the map is displayed in public it can help motivate those households or compounds that have not yet improved their sanitation.

Alternatively it might involve displaying a sticker, coloured rope, or other symbol outside the house to signify that household action has been taken.

When would you use it?	Throughout the process after triggering.

TOOL 5.3 – Institutional performance scoring

What is it?	A method for monitoring the performance of those with responsibility for delivering urban sanitation processes and outcomes, such as ward councillors, other municipal authorities, public health staff, NGO staff, and public or private service providers. This tool should also aim to motivate their active engagement in U-CLTS.
How to use it	Different-coloured cards are used to score the responsible institutional representative against performance in terms of improved sanitation within a particular locality. Red signifies poor performance, yellow shows steady progress, and green indicates good progress. The scorecards are posted against each representative's photograph and displayed in a public place where local residents can see them. This also enhances their accountability. It is important to fully engage with the individuals being scored to explain the scoring method and ensure positive attitudes towards this process. It is also important to acknowledge any difficulties they may be facing and help them to resolve these and improve practice.
Related case studies	Case Study 4: Gulariya, Nepal.

TOOL 5.4 – Community scorecards

What is it?	Local people rank or score the sanitation and hygiene services available to them and are assisted in engaging with service providers and government agencies to discuss the findings and negotiate improvements.
Why use it?	It is an effective means to gain monitoring information relating to service provision as experienced by the users themselves, and translating this information into discussions about improved service provision.

How to use it	Community scorecards should be developed in discussion with community members who identify key issues that form the basis of the indicators to be scored. Once the scorecard is produced, it is rolled out with community members. The scorecard is also used with service providers. This is followed by a meeting between representatives of the community and service providers to discuss the findings and plan actions to address the issues that emerged. The cycle of scoring and reflection can be repeated periodically to ensure that changes are institutionalized.

Challenges associated with community scorecards are that they tend to require a high degree of engagement with different levels of government, and impacts are often 'stuck' at the local level and translate into national-level impacts only where they have plugged into existing reform processes. |
| When would you use it? | This takes place during multiple events over a period of time. |
| Further guidance | CARE Malawi, 2013, http://www.care.org/sites/default/files/documents/FP-2013-CARE_CommunityScoreCardToolkit.pdf

Wild et al., 2015, https://www.odi.org/sites/odi.org.uk/files/odi-assets/publications-opinion-files/9451.pdf |

TOOL 5.5 – Intercommunity monitoring

What is it?	Communities, compounds, or groups monitoring one another to regularly assess progress on sanitation issues.
How to use it	Community or compound representatives are initially brought together to agree a set of monitoring indicators. These might relate to the existence of toilets, their cleanliness, and maintenance of areas within the community or compound. They then make regular visits to one another's community or compound to assess progress against the agreed indicators. This is then reported back at a group meeting to discuss challenges and reasons for slow progress as well as to celebrate and learn from positive outcomes.
Further guidance	Azafady, 2015, www.communityledtotalsanitation.org/sites/communityledtotalsanitation.org/files/Azafady_Adapting_rural_CLTS_for_urban_settings.pdf

TOOL 5.6 – Mobile phone monitoring

What is it?	Mobile phones can be used for data collection for monitoring purposes. Surveys through SMS or other more complex applications are used to collect information on facilities, or on their absence, and can involve geo-tagging locations and photographs of sanitation infrastructure.
Why use it?	Data can be collected quickly and can be made available almost instantaneously, saving a lot of cumbersome paperwork.
How to use it	Various software packages are now available to use with mobile phones in order to collect data on different aspects of sanitation progress. Staff or volunteers can visit households or other locations to collect and input data, including photographs.
	Data collected might include progress towards and completion of toilet construction, existence of handwashing facilities, cleanliness of facilities, maintenance of public spaces (with no OD), etc.
	Data can be uploaded to a computer database, sometimes in real time if relevant connectivity is available. The advantage of mobile phone monitoring is that it reduces paper-based systems, which can be a burden on staff. Data can be entered directly into computer-based systems meaning that it can quickly and easily be analysed and shared, including online. The use of photographs can help overcome misreporting or corruption.
	On the other hand, smartphone-based systems may require technology hardware to be provided by donors. Phones may be lost or stolen or require upgrades, and regular battery recharging may become an issue when using GPS. Software skills are often required, as well as a high degree of backstopping. ICT systems can tend to be extractive rather than community-owned, as the data goes directly to an NGO or government office and community members are unable to access it (Pasteur, 2017).
	There are several examples of the successful use of mobile technologies for monitoring (see Example 5.3). UNICEF Zambia has worked with technical partner Akros to develop an SMS text delivery method that can be used via most basic mobile phones. Community champions collect the data on their own phones and are incentivized to report on time by receiving free talk time when they deliver reports at the end of the month. The data is available on a near real-time basis, with total reporting time from village to national focal points taking 24 hours. On receiving and reviewing the monitoring data, environmental health technicians are able to provide support as necessary.
Further guidance	Pasteur, 2017, http://www.communityledtotalsanitation.org/sites/communityledtotalsanitation.org/files/Keeping_Track_LearningPaper_0.pdf

Nique and Smertnik, 2015, https://www.gsma.com/mobilefordevelopment/wp-content/uploads/2015/08/The-Role-of-Mobile-in-Improved-Sanitation-Access.pdf

UNICEF ESARO, 2015, https://www.unicef.org/esaro/WASH-Field-M2W-low-res.pdf

---

Example 5.3 – Using apps to monitor progress

SeeSaw worked on a U-CLTS project with Practical Action and Umande Trust in Nakuru, Kenya. SeeSaw developed a customized android app that allows local CBOs using low-cost smartphones to record progress in each of 13 'villages' (actually adjoining areas of Nakuru's growing semi-formal settlements). In addition, CBO leaders count the numbers of 'sanitation hotspots' (areas that are not free of OD) and report these regularly, using SeeSaw's 'missed call' system SeeTell. These reports are logged in a central database, mapped, and relayed back to people in Nakuru, who put the numbers up on a physical board in order to report them back to the community itself, an important feedback loop that is too often overlooked.

Source: Pasteur and Prabhakaran, 2015.

Verification, certification, and celebration

The verification, certification, and celebration of goals along the way to a shit-free environment are used to encourage progress and then acknowledge success. They help provide a sense of achievement, which in turn encourages further community-led action. Well-advertised celebrations also raise awareness among neighbouring communities. This process is a hallmark of rural CLTS and has also proved to be successful in the urban context.

In the urban context it can be more difficult. Firstly, a shit-free environment is not a clear goal: alternative goals may be more relevant (see list below). Secondly, one size does not fit all in terms of goals and procedures for measurement, due to the variability of issues across different types of urban context. Thirdly, relevant authorities are currently far less aware of U-CLTS verification and certification processes and therefore protocols and methods do not exist.

Many of the methods for verification and certification are similar to those used for monitoring – i.e. house-to-house visits, community meetings, exchanges, etc. Typically, a verification format will be needed to check off achievements and the standards attained. As there are currently no agreed

U-CLTS goals or criteria for verification, these can generally be generated by communities and relevant partners.

Goals might include the following:

- All available toilets are clean, well maintained, and emptied promptly when full (i.e. none are found to be so full as to be unusable).
- The ratio of toilets to people increases to meet an agreed threshold in the whole community.
- All OD hotspots are cleared and no OD or flying toilets are found.
- Clean public toilets are easily accessible in markets, at bus or train stations, in all schools, health posts, government offices, etc.
- In some peri-urban settings, as a first step it might be appropriate to achieve safe containment in terms of everyone having a toilet.
- Everyone is using safe FSM services.
- FSM service providers are providing safe emptying, transportation, and treatment.

Once the final three goals are achieved (safe containment, safe FSM services, and total usage of these services), total sanitation is achieved.

It is useful for the local authorities to verify and certify, as this will add weight to the achievements and engage the authorities in the issues being addressed. The attitudes of verifiers are very important, as verification should aim to be a form of encouragement.

Multiple verifications help ensure that behaviour change is sustained over time: for example, there could be re-verifications after one, three, and six months, and before certification.

> **Example 5.4 – Encouraging competition between local bodies: *Swachh Survekshan***
>
> The Swachh Bharat Mission (SBM) is the Government of India's national sanitation campaign. As part of the urban programme, the Ministry of Urban Development has commissioned annual *Swachh Survekshan* – a survey and ranking exercise assessing the levels of cleanliness (sanitation and solid and liquid waste management) across different urban local bodies. The goal of the initiative is not only to encourage participation and create awareness but also to incentivize urban bodies to compete to improve service delivery to citizens by ranking highly. Analysis is based on information provided by municipalities, direct observation, and citizen feedback. The results of the ranking are well publicized throughout the media.
>
> The latest survey, conducted in January and February 2018, ranked 434 cities across the country.
>
> *Source*: Government of India, 2018.

TOOL 5.7 – Celebrating progress

What is it?	Organizing celebrations acts as a reward for the community and also generates enthusiasm and commitment among others.
How to use it	Encourage and support communities to celebrate different stages in their progression towards a shit-free environment as well as the final achievement.
	Inviting senior officials, politicians, media, and heads of other communities or administrative units of the same level exposes them to the potential for change. Try to ensure that the VIPs who speak are well informed. Encourage them to invite others to make public statements about progress and plans.
	This involves establishing and agreeing on clear goals or milestones that will be monitored, verified, and celebrated when they are reached.
When would you use it?	After a community has been verified and certified at different stages. It is also useful to organize events for Global Handwashing Day and World Toilet Day (19 November) involving schools, demonstrations, and media coverage.

TOOL 5.8 – Hoarding boards

What is it?	Posters placed in public and community buildings. Large hoarding boards could be placed on roadsides, mainly at junctions, where they would be seen by the maximum number of people.
How to use it	Hoarding boards are produced once a ward becomes a shit-free environment. These boards can serve as a motivating factor for communities that are not yet ODF, as it becomes public knowledge which communities are lagging behind and holding the municipality back from its total sanitation goals. This puts social pressure on those communities to act fast to meet the challenge.

Sustainability

U-CLTS is about engagement and empowerment. Once communities have achieved improved sanitation outcomes, the organizational capacity and enthusiasm already established can be further strengthened to:

- ensure the sustainability of the outcomes – i.e. that there is less chance of slippage over time – through continued monitoring and further upgrading of sanitation technologies;

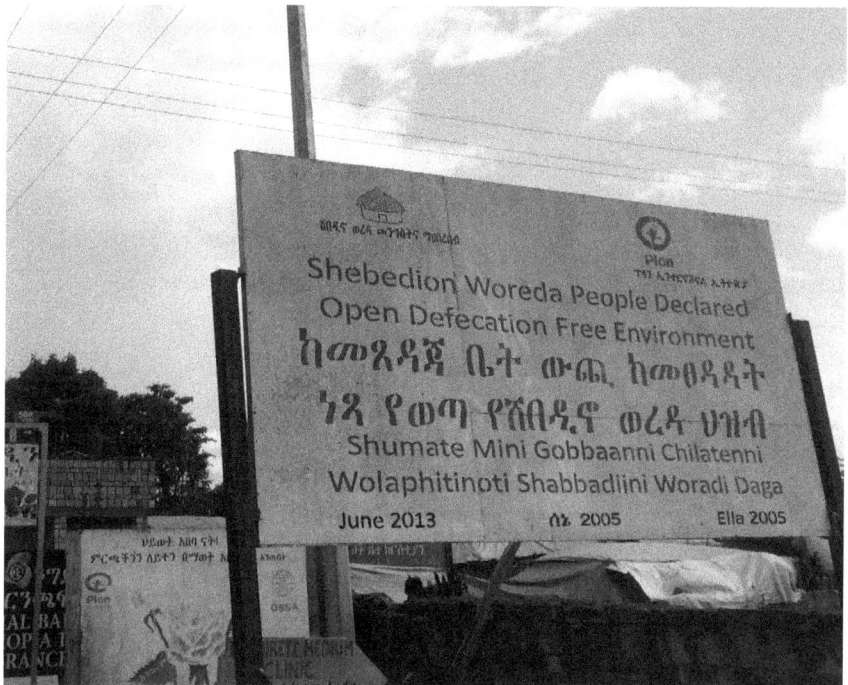

Figure 5.2 Hoarding board in rural town of Shebedion, Ethiopia
Source: Jamie Myers

- address a wider range of issues within the WASH sector – e.g. addressing solid waste, waste water, and general cleanliness of the community; and
- address issues that stretch beyond the sanitation sector, such as housing standards, human rights, employment creation, health and safety, etc.

Similar participatory processes of social mobilization, community-led action, and advocacy can be used to expand the scope of the initial U-CLTS campaign to address wider water- and waste-related issues, such as solid waste, waste water, menstrual hygiene, and a clean environment, as well as human rights, housing, and employment issues. If Natural Leaders and CBOs have been nurtured effectively during U-CLTS, they could be ready to champion other issues.

As noted in Chapter 4, attention should be paid to cultivating sanitation entrepreneurs within communities who will help improve access to sanitation options as a result of their own job opportunities. These might include masons and builders, public toilet businesses, waste collection and sorting enterprises, etc. Such entrepreneurs may require support in developing the relevant skills to be able to manage their business and spread relevant messages.

> **Example 5.5 – Kick-starting a social movement**
>
> Sanitation social movements aim to generate a sense of community identity, dignity, youth mentorship and esteem building, and pride in becoming ODF. A sanitation movement in Nairobi brought together youth groups from different sub-counties across Nairobi County. In Mathare 10, the issue of sanitation was used as a platform for the political claims of marginalized urban dwellers as well as for innovative livelihood strategies for income-poor urban youths: *Usafi ni Power* (Sanitation is Power). The groups met on a monthly basis to deliberate on sanitation issues. The movement's vision was for 'A clean and healthy Nairobi City'. The movement takes part in pre- and post-World Toilet Day clean-up activities. Collaborative effort – including influential and powerful people – is essential to create a social sanitation movement for ODF.
>
> *Source*: Case Study 11, Mathare 10, Nairobi, Kenya; Thieme, 2010.

Dos and don'ts and action points for maintaining momentum

Table 5.1 Dos and don'ts: maintaining momentum

Dos	Don'ts
1. Provide training for Natural Leaders and CBOs to help with follow-up and monitoring activities.	1. Sacrifice speed for quality.
2. Facilitate networking among champions within and between communities and leaders.	2. Stop at the achievement of ODF – Consider using U-CLTS as an entry-point strategy for other community-led development initiatives.
3. Encourage competition between neighbourhoods or settlements.	3. Neglect to support Natural Leaders and CBOs.
4. Celebrate different successes along the way to total sanitation.	4. Set goals that are unattainable and cannot be monitored or verified.
5. If progress is poor, review the whole process to find out what is wrong. This could involve revisiting some of the tools explained in the assessment and preparation section, including scenario planning and political economy analysis.	
6. Work with relevant authorities for verification and certification in an inclusive and participatory manner.	
7. Ensure that there is accountability for commitments from all stakeholders to ensure that gains are maintained.	
8. Plan for frequent follow-up visits and support immediately after triggering and throughout the journey to total sanitation.	
9. Use monitoring visits to identify strengths and challenges and to encourage communities to take doable actions.	

Dos	Don'ts
10. Build a social movement around sanitation.	
11. Document events and outcomes and use these to learn and guide Natural Leaders and communities. Share lessons learned and plan for replication.	

Notes for users

PART 2
Case studies

CHAPTER 6
U-CLTS case studies

Abstract

A U-CLTS approach has been used across different countries in both Africa and Asia. In addition, U-CLTS tools and tactics have also been utilized and integrated into wider sanitation programmes. The focus of Part 2 is 'how others have done it' – 15 different case studies are presented outlining the different contexts, objectives, good practices, and challenges of each intervention. The purpose is to draw inspiration from others' learning and from both what went well and what went wrong.

Keywords: U-CLTS; case studies; sanitation programmes; U-CLTS tools; U-CLTS tactics; urban sanitation.

Introduction to the case studies

This part provides a description of 15 case studies. They are given to show 'how others have done it'. The point is not for people to copy and paste these examples but for them to find inspiration and ideas. Each case study highlights good practice and lessons learned as well as previous and current challenges. The studies are:

1. Choma, Zambia
2. Eight towns in Ethiopia
3. Fort Dauphin, Madagascar
4. Gulariya, Nepal
5. Hawassa, Ethiopia
6. Himbirti, Eritrea
7. Iringa, Tanzania
8. IUWASH, Indonesia
9. Kabwe, Zambia
10. Logo, Nigeria
11. Mathare 10, Nairobi, Kenya
12. Nakuru, Kenya
13. New Delhi, India,
14. Ribaué and Rapale, Mozambique
15. Small towns in Northern and Southern Nigeria

These cases come from a range of different countries and urban typologies. They have not been written by the authors of Part 1 but by those who have been involved in the programmes, projects, and interventions they describe. Interventions date back to 2006 and many of the case studies use rural terminologies.

The case studies have been standardized where appropriate. They focus on good practice, challenges, and lessons learned.

We expect this section to grow over time and we encourage people to document their experiences – including both failures and successes – and to share them with us via CLTS@ids.ac.uk. Future case studies will be made available at http://www.communityledtotalsanitation.org/Innovations-for-Urban-Sanitation-casestudies.

Case Study 1: Choma, Zambia

Giveson Zulu, Wash Specialist, UNICEF Zambia

Context	The Choma Joint Monitoring Programme Team (JMPT) for sanitation implemented CLTS in peri-urban and urban areas of Choma District.
Implementing organization	UNICEF
Objectives	To ensure adequate sanitation in institutions, public places, and tenant households as specified in the Zambian Public Health Act.
Description of good practices	Initial attempts had limited success, especially in the most urbanized settings, because of the predominance of tenant households, the high population density, and weaker community structures. Consequently, the JMPT decided to adapt CLTS for urban areas to complement the continued CLTS programme in rural areas with a programme of legal enforcement in urban and peri-urban areas. Details are listed below.

- The legal enforcement uses the '3 rope approach': technocrats, civic leaders, and the judiciary (who replaced the role of traditional rulers used in rural CLTS). Its focus is on landlords and public and private institutions.
- The legal enforcement approach is a strategy initiated to address and confront 'urban nuisances' related to sanitation as well as food and general hygiene. U-CLTS (legal enforcement) was implemented initially as an emergency preparedness strategy and a response to cholera outbreaks in Lusaka, targeting the most affected areas. Training sessions were held in other districts to sensitize the business community, government, and public on adhering to public health and food safety laws.
- The specific targets of CLTS legal enforcement are:
  - public places;
  - public buildings (i.e. government buildings, schools);
  - food establishments; and
  - lodges, etc.
- Extensive networks to coordinate CLTS programming have been developed at the national level (through a national CLTS team), district (through the development of the JMPT), urban and peri-urban (legal enforcement groups or LEGs), and rural (sanitation action groups).

The legal enforcement approach follows the following steps:

1. *Field preparations and field work.* It is important to ensure that everybody gets a chance to go into the field to experience first-hand the gravity of the problem within their locality and the need for a concerted effort for everyone to work together for meaningful change.
2. *Triggering.* Where the groups go to the communities to sensitize them on what is being and what can be done and to find out what they want to do.
3. *Way forward/action planning.* A legal enforcement work plan for two months.
4. *Post-triggering.* This includes prosecution, monitoring and evaluation, and reporting.
5. *Prosecution process.* Preparation of notices and summons of non-compliant people or premises.
6. *Monitoring (follow-up).* To check compliance and spend time educating citizens.

	7. *Mid-term evaluation*. A review of progress after one month from the triggering and preparation for evaluation. 8. *Evaluation workshop*. A review of trigger reports, the action plan, and stakeholder participation, and updating the database.
Challenges	In peri-urban areas, over 40% of households did not have toilets. In addition: • Many people in the peri-urban areas are tenants (about 50%) and they could not build toilets without their landlord's permission (this is why public health laws had to be enforced). • Whether the toilets are built by the tenants or the landlords, there is a greater possibility of the house rent going up, hence creating a double-bind situation for the tenants. • The timing of triggering is difficult as the household heads are usually at work during the day in the week, which means that flexibility is needed.
Results	• People started demanding sanitation and handwashing facilities at health centres. • Public institutions and food-vending locations are now targets of sanitation orders, and there are examples where the public has taken out orders against local authorities, bars, restaurants, or schools to construct sanitation facilities. • People call in to radio programmes and report or complain about institutions that do not have sanitation facilities.
Lessons	• Pre-triggering emphasis on understanding **power relationships and leadership** in the local context helped create an in-depth understanding of how people at the local level are influenced. There are also possibilities for involving other groups such as influential area development commissions or NGOs. • **Longer-term support** (training and networking) is needed for public health officials or environmental health technologists (EHTs) from the district council or district public health, and for LEGs. Support is needed for EHTs to monitor progress on, for example, transport, fuel, and continuous capacity building, particularly when they are conducting follow-up. As EHTs/public health officers or Community Health Workers can be the link to communities in reinforcing CLTS, support is needed over the long term, especially where they are supporting LEGs. • The CLTS coordinating bodies should have diverse representation, i.e. from health, legal enforcement, media, NGOs, and the judiciary.
References	Zulu, G. (2011) *Urban CLTS in Zambia: The Case of Choma and Lusaka*, UNICEF Zambia, Lusaka, http://www.communityledtotalsanitation.org/resource/urban-clts-zambia [accessed 25 February 2018].

Case Study 2: Eight towns in Ethiopia

Abiyou Worku Yohannes, Regional WASH Coordinator, World Vision Ethiopia

Context	CLTS was implemented in eight towns and 26 satellite villages with a combined population of 100,000. It also covered 21 health institutions and 98 schools. The eight towns were: • Sheno, Abomsa, and Wolenchity, Oromia Region; • Maksegnit, Amhara Region; • Wukro and Adheshu, Tigray; and • Kebridehar and Jigjiga, Somali Region.
Implementing organizations	UNICEF and World Vision Ethiopia (WVE).
Funding details	Total agreed budget of US$2,691,802.
Objectives	• Strengthened governance systems for equitable, effective, and transparent WASH resource allocation through the promotion and monitoring of equity and social accountability in delivering WASH services (these are defined as: water, sanitation, hygiene, and liquid and solid waste management services) both at national and programme level. • Enhanced capacity of the Consortium of Christian Relief and Development Associations' Water and Sanitation Forum (WSF) to coordinate civil society organizations within Ethiopia's WASH sector for the implementation of the ONE WASH national programme (OWNP). • Development of a comprehensive hygiene and environmental sanitation promotion package to increase the sustainable use of WASH facilities, services, and products at household and community level. • Capacity-building resources developed to enhance understanding of OWNP and WASH provision in Ethiopia.
Dates	The project finished in June 2017.
Sanitation solutions	• The community built their own toilets. • UNICEF built public latrines in densely populated areas and for the most vulnerable communities.
Description of good practices	• The programme focused on: ODF towns and satellite villages, institutional WASH, menstrual hygiene management, capacity building of WASH service providers and partners, hygiene promotion, and waste management. • Sanitation Master Plans were developed for all the eight towns in the programme. Open WASH modules were developed for vocational and technical colleges and training was also provided. Four manuals were developed for health extension workers, public–private operators, artisans, parent–teacher associations, school directors, and school club members. Training was also given to the respective target groups to facilitate waste management, the production of sanitation technologies, and institutional WASH as part of activities carried out successfully under this function. In 2016, close to 1,000 people took part in the capacity-building training, with the aim of strengthening their respective institutions and working to improve urban WASH. • The social accountability promoted by the World Vision 'Citizen Voice of Action' programme addressed the most vulnerable groups. This tool

facilitates dialogue among stakeholders through a series of interactive processes that enable every participant to actively engage and contribute to the development of an action plan based on identified problems and suggested solutions. The dialogue processes involved setting minimum WASH service standards, visiting service locations to observe the prevailing situation compared with the agreed standards, providing feedback (scorecard approach), and designing a joint action plan based on consideration of the needs of the most vulnerable groups.

- The joint action plans provide a clear framework of accountability on who is responsible for what services, when to undertake service delivery, and how monitoring is to be done. Key participants in these forums include *kebele* representatives, health extension workers, officials of the municipalities, and organized *ketena* sanitation and hygiene taskforces.

Results

Urban ODF is challenging, especially in developing countries such as Ethiopia. Currently, World Vision in collaboration with its partners (UNICEF and DFID) is implementing a pilot urban WASH project. World Vision integrated Community Voice of Action into the CLTS tools. The result was that eight *ketenas* (the smallest administration unit) were declared ODF. The practice of OD is becoming history in these towns. The project was successful and provides many lessons for WASH practitioners. Lessons include the importance of integrating Community Voice of Action into CLTSH (CLTS + Hygiene) and through the 1-5 Development Army (a network of women volunteers found across Ethiopia), and the alignment of CLTS with enforcement of sanitation by-laws.

Integrating CLTSH with Community Voice of Action helped towns become ODF more quickly and increased communication among the community. It also resulted in the following:

- More household latrines were constructed.
- More hygiene and sanitation mass campaigns were organized by communities.
- Community environmental cleaning campaigns were better attended.
- Sanitation ambassadors and organized taskforces encouraged neighbouring communities to implement urban CLTS and adopt safe hygiene practices.
- There was more condemnation of OD practices in communities.

These activities were supported by more rigorous verification, feedback, and intensified follow-up activities to support the town *ketenas* that attained ODF status.

Lessons

1. Community Voice of Action led to the inclusion of vulnerable communities in the implementation of U-CLTS.
2. Communities were involved in innovative latrine construction in flood-prone areas.
3. U-CLTS needs government and political commitment, enforcement, and the involvement of more stakeholders.
4. Use of the existing government platforms yields more results in urban ODF processes.

References

World Vision Ethiopia (n.d.) 'The urban WASH field reports, August 2014–2017', unpublished report.

Case Study 3: Fort Dauphin, Madagascar

Rachel Hammersley-Mather, Head of Project Development, SEED Madagascar

Context	Project Malio worked with households, communities, and institutions to improve sanitation and hygiene in Fort Dauphin, a medium-sized town (85,000) with peri-urban areas. CLTS activities were used to challenge OD practices in communities in particular.
Implementing organizations	SEED Madagascar and ONG Azafady.
Funding details	Big Lottery Fund (£374,067) and Guernsey Overseas Aid and Development Commission (£58,443).
Objectives	1. Town-wide uptake of community action plans to reduce the practice of OD and institutionalize positive hygiene practices, leading to improved health across the community. 2. Increased number of household latrines and motivation regarding their use and maintenance, leading to a reduction in the practice of OD and subsequent diarrhoeal disease at the household level. 3. Increased number of school latrines and motivation regarding their use and maintenance among the town's children, reducing the practice of OD and diarrhoeal disease in those most vulnerable to hygiene-related illnesses. 4. A communal latrine is operational with sustainable cleaning and maintenance mechanisms, thereby increasing access for overcrowded households, reducing contamination of local water sources, and improving health among the most disadvantaged.
Dates	May 2014–April 2017. The project is now closed; however, a new project to address FSM requirements for sanitation facilities is currently being developed.
Sanitation solutions	• Ventilated improved pit (VIP) latrines for households. • A septic tank at one community latrine. • A variety of sanitation facilities built or refurbished at 11 schools.
Description of good practices	Key activities included: • construction support for 799 household latrines and 11 school latrine blocks; • training and mentorship for six local associations; • support for local authorities, including sector-level action-planning sessions; and • town-wide mass mobilizations and high-profile multimedia campaigns.
Challenges	Malio encountered numerous challenges in its application of CLTS in an urban setting including: • Triggering was condensed to a single morning and omitted key activities such as transect walks due to sectors lacking defined borders. The lack of borders provided a ready excuse for residents to blame other members of the large community for the filth in their own neighbourhood. • Key messages often lost impact due to the inability of triggerings to occur simultaneously across the wider community. For example, demonstrations including 'shit–fly–food' and 'shit calculations' lost shock value as more people were exposed to Malio messages ahead of triggering. • CLTS facilitates immediate action to improve sanitation, but as the project progressed and people recognized the opportunity for subsidized latrines, motivation was reduced in households hoping to be eligible for a latrine.

Challenges linked to latrine emptying included the following:

- Vulnerable households who are unable to otherwise afford latrines may find it difficult to prioritize latrine maintenance and the cost of ongoing emptying, particularly in an environment where sustained financial management is not engrained.
- Latrines are likely to fill very quickly due to high usage, with some neighbourhoods averaging almost 20 users per latrine.
- While focus groups covered safe emptying procedures, even the poorest households may not be inclined to empty latrines independently due to the stigma attached.
- Full, unemptied latrines had a detrimental impact on sustained behaviour change, with people reverting to OD rather than emptying latrines.

Other challenges included the following:

- Motivated community leaders frequently suggested fining people caught openly defecating but were unable to do so, due to community groups' inability to implement these fines independently and a lack of municipal enforcement.
- Hygiene promotion remains a challenge in Fort Dauphin due to intermittent water supply, with most households and many institutions, including schools, lacking mains water.

Results

Overall, approximately 18,000 people benefited through sanitation provision at household and school levels.

Outcome 1

- 10 community action plans were developed and implemented across 10 Fort Dauphin *fokontany* (districts).
- 98% of respondents to a random community survey ($n = 500$) reported washing their hands before eating and after defecating.
- 436 households outside Malio's triggering zones requested help to construct a latrine.

Outcome 2

- 799 household latrines were constructed, and 799 households actively participated in support groups.
- 274 households emptied latrines as a direct result of the project (85% of all project latrines that had filled).
- There was an 85% reduction in beneficiary children under five suffering from chronic diarrhoea, and a 23% increase in beneficiary children never having diarrhoea.

Outcome 3

- 17 schools were supported by Malio to develop and implement sanitation action plans, with 11 schools achieving 'Friend of WASH' status.
- 11 schools are using and maintaining improved sanitation facilities.
- 9,139 students engaged in mass mobilizations, while 6,567 participated in WASH education sessions.
- A commune-wide school WASH committee monitors school WASH outcomes.

Outcome 4

- A public latrine was refurbished, with an average of 78 users per day and a consistently high score for cleanliness.
- Pay-for-use covers the guardian and ongoing cleaning fee.
- Competitions between households triggers sectors and rewards those who have made most progress.

Lessons	- Ongoing capacity building motivates the team and enhances confidence when sharing thoughts and learning, as they know their feedback informs project adaptations and decisions.
- Research into appropriate FSM options should occur simultaneously with other project activities, with emerging challenges tied into the FSM response.
- When working with staff who have prior experience of triggering, it is helpful to learn which activities they use and what style of facilitation is preferred; as a team, agree on guidelines and standards to ensure consistency.
- As front-line staff engaging with beneficiary households, it is essential for construction staff to also have a sound working knowledge of CLTS.
- Ahead of their use, households sharing latrines should be encouraged to agree on management and maintenance arrangements to avoid disputes about cleaning and emptying once they begin to fill.
- Mass media campaigns, including radio broadcasts and signboards with very visual messages, are extremely useful for sharing project messages, hosting debates, and exploring key concepts with low-literacy populations.
- The application of CLTS should be carefully considered alongside local team members in communities with traditional taboos around discussions of faeces, and in small communities where team members may feel extreme discomfort due to the potential offence caused to friends, neighbours, and elders.
- CLTS activities can challenge team members within the organization.
References	SEED Madagascar (2017) *Final Report for Project Malio: A Community-led Approach to Eliminating OD and Facilitating Sustained Behaviour Change*, London, SEED Madagascar, https://madagascar.co.uk/application/files/8515/0461/2575/Project_Malio_Final_Report_July_2017.pdf [accessed 25 February 2018].

Case Study 4: Gulariya, Nepal

Lucy Stevens, Senior Policy and Practice Adviser, Practical Action
Based on Pasteur et al. 2016

Context	Gulariya municipality, Bardiya district, south-western Nepal, is divided into 14 wards and 243 *toles* (communities), with a total population of 60,379 (10,922 households). The municipality is a mix of settlement types, with about 15% urban/small towns and the remaining 85% peri-urban (at the interface between rural and urban zones, activities, and services). It has a fast-growing population due to inward migration.
Implementing organizations	Practical Action Nepal and Environmental and Public Health Organization.
Funding details	£200,000 from DFID (under an Aid Match grant).
Objectives	Achieving ODF status in the remaining 11 wards in Gulariya municipality, with six wards to achieve 'total sanitation' status. Project planned outputs were: • increased coverage of sanitation facilities so that the entire municipality is ODF; • enhanced capacity for stakeholders; • piloting of innovative solutions in sanitation to improve disaster-resilient sanitation facilities and FSM; and • promotion of inclusive and good governance through a participatory planning approach.
Dates	August 2014–July 2016 (24 months in total).
Sanitation solutions	• Over 90% constructed offset, lined, ventilated pit latrines. • Fewer than 5% constructed septic tanks. • A couple of examples of biogas toilets constructed with the support of a government subsidy.
Description of good practices	**Pre-triggering** in communities began with the orientation and training of Ward WASH Coordination Committees (W-WASH-CCs) and other institutional actors. During the W-WASH-CC orientation, plans were drawn up for the process of entering each of 186 *toles* within the 11 wards that were not yet ODF. Pre-triggering activities involved meeting with key actors within the *tole*, including Tole Lane Organization (TLO) committee members, *badaghars* (social leaders), religious leaders, etc. The meeting was facilitated by one or two members of the W-WASH-CC, a member of the Municipality Water Supply, Sanitation, and Hygiene Coordination Committee (M-WASH-CC), and project staff. Additionally, the following activities were conducted: • baseline survey to identify toilet coverage of the municipality (11 wards); • feeding back information on sanitation status to TLOs, W-WASH-CCs, M-WASH-CC, District Water Supply, Sanitation, and Hygiene Coordination Committee (D-WASH-CC), and political parties; and • activating and orienting local institutions (TLOs, mothers' groups, Female Community Health Volunteers (FCHVs), WatSan (water and sanitation) volunteers, W-WASH-CCs, child clubs, etc.). Various strategies were employed for **triggering** in communities depending on the nature of the intended intervention and the extent of OD in the communities, in order to achieve wider development goals: • The initial entry point was a community discussion and video shows. • Communities were mobilized for triggering.

- Triggering tools and processes included the creation of a community map; mapping of typical OD sites; illustration of faecal–oral contamination routes, including the 'food and soda' exercise; shit calculation; calculation of medical expenses; whistle campaign.
- Institutional triggering was conducted with the project management committee (PMC), M-WASH-CC, W-WASH-CCs, TLOs, and citizen awareness centres.
- Triggering was conducted through informal/non-governmental structures (FCHVs, mothers' groups, WatSan volunteers, *badaghars*, child clubs, etc.).

For **post-triggering follow-up**, techniques applied included: door-to-door campaigns; street drama; showing a film called *Charpi Bihe*; using hoardings and posters; the municipality issuing a sanitation card and other service-based incentives; *tole*-level fines; social pressure (through W-WASH-CCs, TLOs, FCHVs, WatSan volunteers, *badaghars*, mothers' groups, religious leaders, neighbours, child clubs, etc.). Some of these tools could be considered for ongoing repeated triggering. In fact, facilitators often returned to communities to use CLTS tools if the initial triggering was not effective.

Post-ODF activities supported by the project can be divided into two groups. Firstly, the project carries out a regular meeting of W-WASH-CCs in all 14 wards, preparing action plans and mobilizing them for regular monitoring/follow-up. Secondly, the project worked in six ODF communities (22 TLOs out of a total of 243) to achieve 'total sanitation', which involves achieving a number of further hygiene- and sanitation-related targets.

The project is piloting FSM, which is needed urgently to address the problem of the filling-up of toilets. This is a public–private partnership between the municipality and a local company and involved local composting of faecal sludge. The project is considering ways to support informal manual pit emptiers to ensure a diversity of safe and hygienic emptying options for the local population.

Challenges
- Internal migration brings in people to urban areas with different cultures and languages as well as varying knowledge and practice on WASH, which keeps a rolling challenge to maintain ODF status.
- Due to soaring land prices and unaffordability, a significant segment of people in urban areas reside in rented properties and are reluctant to invest in building toilets.
- Limited space in some slum/squatter settlements poses problems in constructing individual toilets (shared toilets pose a challenge of proper operation and maintenance and are not popular or widely promoted in Nepal).
- Some households could afford only a shallow lined pit that fills up quickly – investment is now being made in pit emptying and safe disposal services, but it would have been more economical in the long term to find ways to help families dig a deeper pit.

Results
- Around 5,385 toilets were built to a high standard.
- ODF status was declared in May 2015. ODF status was achieved with the construction of individual toilets, 319 institutional toilets, and five public toilets.

- A population of over 30,000 were engaged who were practising OD.
- Out of 14 wards within Gulariya municipality, the project facilitated achieving ODF in 11 wards within a six-month time period.
- Two communities declared 'total sanitation' status requiring: toilets and their proper use; safe drinking water; safe hygiene practices; food hygiene and clean kitchens; and clean household environments.
- Existing government structures have been used positively to support urban (and rural) CLTS processes. In some cases it may be mandatory to work through such structures (as in Practical Action's experience in Nepal).

Lessons

- Since urban communities are heterogeneous, CLTS and household-centred approaches should be combined for better effect.
- In addition to local/Natural Leaders, local institutions play a crucial role in creating local pressure and sustaining ODF. Without institutional buy-in and commitment, efforts to support ODF communities can be short-lived. Institutional triggering can be considered a significant element of the U-CLTS approach.
- Priority should be given to women attending the triggering meetings because they understand the issues better and then they would pressure their husbands to build a toilet and educate their children around behaviour change.
- Involving government and local authorities from the start will also help ensure that U-CLTS processes fit into and complement existing frameworks and plans.
- Systematic, regular, and multi-institutional follow-up immediately after triggering was key to achieving ODF in a short period of time. The many messages and pressures coming from all sides to improve sanitation achieved swift impact.

References

Pasteur, K. and Prabhakaran, P. with Kar, K. (2016) *Achieving Open Defecation Free Gulariya Municipality*, Kolkata, CLTS Foundation, http://www.cltsfoundation.org/wp-content/uploads/2017/03/Gulariya-Municipality_Nepal_CLTS-Foundation_Practical-Action.pdf [accessed 9 November 2017].

Project website: https://practicalaction.org/safa.

Series of blogs on the project: https://practicalaction.org/blog/?s=gulariya.

Case Study 5: Hawassa, Ethiopia

Gashaw Kebede, WASH Programme Lead, Plan International Ethiopia

Context	Hawassa is a small- to medium-sized town and the capital of the Southern Nations, Nationalities, and Peoples Regional State, Ethiopia. The population of the town is 25,861, with the number living in the project slums being 11,566.
Implementing organizations	An 11-month project was funded by Plan International Ethiopia and coordinated by Nazareth Children's Village Integrated Development (NACID).
Funding details	Funded by Plan Netherlands. Total budget was 608,252 Ethiopian Birr (US$31,896). Including the additional funds allocated by the municipality, the total for the project was approximately 1,000,000 Ethiopian Birr (US$52,439).
Objectives	To test CLTS tools and processes in the urban context.
Dates	The project lasted for 11 months in 2013–14
Sanitation solutions	• Community latrines; • Pit latrines; • Cleaning dirty toilets; • Improving existing toilets; • Increasing the number of toilets per compound.
Description of good practices	• The project was trying to tackle OD, dirty toilets, and the dumping of solid and liquid waste. • Twenty 'urban slum villages' were selected with the municipality – which also signed off on the project. • It was not 100% subsidy-free – people without space or resources had public and communal toilets built for them. • Pre-triggering community meetings were held in each slum village and people were asked to elect someone to join a community facilitation team. The team members were then given five days' CLTS training and conducted the triggering. • During community triggering, shit calculations were adapted to include shit that was dumped into the environment – thus including flying toilets. They also included solid waste calculations. Pathways for faecal contamination and transect walks were successful; however, mapping exercises were found to be too time-consuming. In areas where different households live together in compounds, household/compound triggering took place. Each compound was visited and household triggering was conducted. This involved facilitating discussions on sanitation and solid and liquid waste. Instead of going to OD areas, households were taken to the compound toilets. Household/compound triggering was used as a post-triggering activity and was effective at reaching households that did not attend community triggering. • Natural Leaders emerging from CLTS triggering were given training to conduct household/compound triggering. They were also provided with carts, boots, and gloves to collect rubbish, thus generating income for themselves. Natural Leaders were encouraged to form community-based entrepreneur groups (CBEs) that collected rubbish and could eventually empty latrines.

Challenges	• ODF was not achieved and is still a challenge in certain communities.
• There is a lack of solid waste management. Natural Leader groups were promised a site for the rubbish collected but it was too far away to be accessible by cart.
• Toilets for street dwellers and communal latrines for those with little space are not sufficient in either number or quality.
• Problems remain with some of the communal latrines that were built and there is little sense of ownership.
Results	• A U-CLTS guide was written by Plan International Ethiopia.
• Plan International Ethiopia worked with government health extension workers who are already delivering sanitation and hygiene messages at the household level to implement U-CLTS.
• Plan International Ethiopia worked with government to ensure that solid waste management, beautification, or other relevant municipality priorities were integrated into ODF targets. This is a way of raising the priority of sanitation within government or the authorities.
• Local governments agreed to provide land for CBEs to use to dump solid waste they collected from communities; however, the space should be appropriate.
Lessons	• The approach in Hawassa was adapted using lessons learned during the implementation of CLTS in Leku Town and Manicho.
• Involving local governments helps ensure that support (for follow-up and monitoring) is available for Natural Leaders post-triggering. However, working with local government can also slow down the process.
• There should be an urban sanitation strategy or urban ODF protocol from central government.
References	Myers, J. (2016) *Plan Netherlands' Experience of Using a CLTS Approach in Urban Environments*, Amsterdam, Plan Nederland, http://www.communityledtotalsanitation.org/sites/communityledtotalsanitation.org/files/Urban_CLTS_Plan.pdf [accessed 5 September 2016].

Case Study 6: Himbirti, Eritrea

Yirgalem Solomon, WASH Specialist, UNICEF Eritrea

Context	Himbirti community is located around 30 km north of the Eritrean capital of Asmara. With a population of 11,000, it was the first large peri-urban community to be declared ODF in Eritrea. The majority of the population were practising OD and the demand for sanitation was extremely low, with just 10% of the households having access to their own toilet.
Implementing organizations	The Ministry of Health, Environmental Health Division in collaboration with the Maekel region Environmental Health Division. UNICEF Eritrea provided technical and financial support to the project. The CLTS facilitators were Ministry of Health and local public health officers.
Funding details	Funded by UNICEF.
Objectives	ODF Himbirti.
Dates	2009–12.
Overview	*Triggering tools used.* Transect walk (OD mapping); shit and food; shit and water; shit calculations; medical expense calculations. *ODF criteria.* Availability and use of latrines, availability of soap/ash and water next to latrine, environmental cleanliness, knowledge of improved sanitation/hygiene practices (verified by asking test questions). **A 'damp matchbox'** The initial triggering of Himbirti was conducted in June 2009, with very poor results. Only around 150 people attended the triggering session (around 1% of the population) and, after one year, only one member of the community had constructed a latrine. On reflection, many mistakes were made. The time spent in pre-triggering of the town was minimal; it was assumed that just a few short visits to a handful of the community leaders would be sufficient to secure their commitment to CLTS and mobilize the rest of the community. It was also assumed the messages conveyed during triggering demonstrations would be automatically disseminated to the rest of the community, as had often been the case in rural communities. Unfortunately, the triggering did not generate the same enthusiasm experienced in rural communities, despite using the triggering techniques. **Promising flames** The 're-triggering' of Himbirti occurred in 2010. Government staff returned to Himbirti, determined to learn from past mistakes and rally together to ensure that this time the entire community could be declared ODF. Several critical adaptations were made to the CLTS process to make it more suitable for peri-urban areas.
Challenges and descriptions of good practices	**Pre-triggering** Challenge 1: Winning over town leaders in the pre-triggering process is vital in order to gain genuine enthusiasm and support for the CLTS process. The second time around, the facilitators focused on the engagement of key town leaders, including, most importantly, the administrator. Members of the local government health team organized several advocacy workshops at the community level for leaders (including health staff, community group leaders, and religious leaders). In addition,

numerous one-on-one sessions were also held with the administrator and other leaders, with support from the Ministry of Health. Support from the zonal administrator and sub-zonal administrators were also vital in the engagement and motivation of town officials. This support had been generated several months previously via similar one-on-one meetings and advocacy workshops, led by the Ministry of Health and local government (*zoba*) health teams. As a result, the zonal and sub-zonal administrators were now highly supportive of CLTS. The Ministry of Health also actively helped promote competition between zonal and sub-zonal administrators, recognizing those who were achieving results at national events and workshops, in addition to inviting those who were not as successful to ODF certification exercises and ceremonies.

Challenge 2: Ensuring the whole town attended triggering. Once key leaders were mobilized, they worked alongside health workers to mobilize the entire town. This took several weeks, with special effort being made to ensure that community members were informed well in advance of the triggering dates. As a result, around 80% to 90% of the population attended the triggering sessions.

Triggering

Challenge 1: Population constraints. The sheer size of Himbirti meant that it was impractical to trigger the entire community all at once. Instead, the town was divided up into three zones, and then into clusters of 50 households – each cluster was then assigned a CLTS facilitator from the local health centre. The triggering of clusters took place over a two-day period with neighbouring clusters being triggered simultaneously wherever possible. Following triggering, each cluster then generated at least one Natural Leader who was then responsible for motivating and monitoring their respective clusters. At least 60% of Himbirti's Natural Leaders are women.

Challenge 2: Demand for expensive latrines. A previous history of subsidy, in addition to community wealth divisions, meant that around 10% of households already had latrines and therefore felt somewhat exempt from the triggering process. Several of these community members were reported as being 'disruptive' during triggering, vocally demanding subsidies and high-quality latrines (made from cement and imported materials) as opposed to those made from 'cheap local materials' (such as wood and mud). Status and pride were obviously very important motivators for behaviour change within Himbirti, and were therefore harnessed by facilitators during the triggering process. Facilitators worked extensively with community members to discuss desirable options, particularly for those who couldn't afford cement and imported materials. Examples were given of attractive improved latrines, made from wood/mud superstructures with plastic or mud slabs. Community members were assured that these were 'just as good' as cement latrines, and they were something to be proud of, with examples being given from neighbouring communities. This was something that was also supported by the administrator and religious leaders. Communities also received construction guidelines from the Ministry of Health, including recommendations on the depth of pits to help ensure quality construction.

Post-triggering

Challenge 1: Hard rock. This means that digging a pit can often become a laborious and time-consuming process involving the softening of soil (in stages) by using water. One pit can therefore take many weeks to dig. To overcome this challenge many community members instead opted to dig pits around 1.5 metres deep and raise the foundations to create 'Everest latrines', guided by the support of the CLTS facilitators and Natural Leaders.

Challenge 2: Termites. The insects destroy any wood used in construction, including that which is used to support the slab, leading to the collapse of the latrine. Local innovations to combat termites have included painting burnt (recycled) oil or salt onto the wood. Facilitators and Natural Leaders also encourage families to start using their latrines immediately following construction in addition to using tight-fitting latrine covers that deter the termites from settling in the latrine.

Challenge 3: Space constraints. Many neighbouring households decided to come together and jointly dig a larger shared pit with two separate superstructures (one for each family). Foundations were also raised to create more depth.

Challenge 4: Property rental and new settlers. In Himbirti, health centres monitor the completion and maintenance of latrines, as is the case for all other CLTS communities across Eritrea. Once a latrine has been certified by the health centre, the family will receive a confirmation slip that is then stapled into the front of their personal file which resides with the town administrator. This process helps serve as an incentive for new community members, who receive a file on arrival, to construct latrines. Key ministry officials are therefore advocating for legislation that demands mandatory inclusion of toilets in all rental properties, with the tenant being responsible for maintenance. This would be enforced at the *zoba* level and would complement any existing bans on OD, which many community and town administrators have decided to impose.

Maintaining ODF status

Challenge 1: Ensuring sustained monitoring post-ODF. Extensive monitoring by a mixture of actors (health staff, Natural Leaders, women's associations, sub-*zoba* taskforces, *zoba* government health officers and Ministry of Health) has been vital in ensuring long-term behaviour change and retention of ODF status.

Challenge 2: Handwashing. Almost one year after the town was declared ODF, many households still do not have soap and water next to their latrine. If washing hands takes place elsewhere in the household, many people reportedly just use water. Plastic jerry cans were initially used by many households but reports of 'children moving them' and 'rats eating the soap' meant that many handwashing facilities have since been removed. The Ministry of Health/UNICEF provided handwashing facilities (in the form of a water storage container with a tap) for a select number of people in the community (those who have the fastest or best constructed latrines) as part of the ODF celebrations.

Challenge 3: Ensuring the spread of CLTS to neighbouring communities. Promoting competition and advocating for CLTS support at the *zoba* and sub-*zoba* levels has been critical in ensuring the spread of CLTS across Eritrea. The Ministry of Health actively encourages this by advocating with local government partners, holding experience-sharing workshops and arranging learning trips between *zobas*. At the community level, health workers and Natural Leaders continue to spread the word and trigger neighbouring communities (without the direct support of a facilitator). Inviting non-ODF administrators, religious leaders, and community members to attend ODF verification exercises and ODF ceremonies has also helped encourage the spread of CLTS. In fact, two large towns neighbouring Himbirti recently commenced CLTS, largely as a result of the town's ODF ceremony in 2012. Several administrators reportedly took exception to the fact that they were asked to sit behind members of the ODF community and did not receiving accolades during the event. Signboards, supported by the Ministry of Health, are also placed in prominent locations to help enforce community pride and ensure accountability for their ODF status – in addition to encouraging their neighbours to follow suit.

Results Himbirti town was declared ODF in February 2012. People from across the region attended the celebrations, including the Governor, Minister of Health, *zoba* and sub-*zoba* administrators, and religious and community leaders from neighbouring towns and villages.

Lessons
- U-CLTS has the potential to be one of the best methods of achieving rapid and sustainable use of improved sanitation at scale.
- Strong government leadership, quality facilitation (including the segmentation of larger populations) and constant monitoring are important prerequisites for CLTS to be successful in rural communities and have been found to be absolutely essential for peri-urban CLTS.
- Breaking up the community into small segments proved beneficial.
- Lack of space to build latrines was overcome by the sharing of pits but not the superstructure.
- It is important to advocate for legislation that makes it mandatory for all rental properties to have a toilet.

References Solomon, Y. (2013) *CLTS in Himbirti, Asmara, Eritrea*, UNICEF Eritrea, Asmara, http://www.communityledtotalsanitation.org/resource/achieving-odf-peri-urban-settings-clts-himbirti [accessed 25 February 2018].

Case Study 7: Iringa, Tanzania

Samson Maswaga, Project Officer, MAMADO and Jörg Henkel, Project Manager, Fondazione ACRA

Context	A Community-Led Urban Environmental Sanitation (CLUES) project has been implemented in five low-density/peri-urban wards in Iringa municipality, Tanzania, where CLTS triggering tools were used.
	The ward has 13,266 households. The target was that at least 20% of households would attend a CLUES workshop and 2,650 households were expected to be reached through CLUES.
Implementing organizations	Fondazione ACRA and Maji na Maendeleo Dodoma (MAMADO).
Funding details	Funded by the European Union. Total project cost is €1,834,509 over five years. €19,969 was spent on the CLUES workshop.
Objectives	Health and hygiene conditions of poor communities living in peri-urban Iringa municipality are improved, with great attention given to environmental, social, and economic sustainability of implemented solutions.
Dates	Ongoing. As of February 2018, the project was ending its fourth project year and entering its fifth and final year.
Sanitation solutions	• Pour-flush toilets. • Raised Fossa Alterna – an alternating double-pit system. Waste is transformed into a nutrient-rich soil conditioner. When one pit is full it is left to decompose while the other is used. • Decentralized wastewater treatment system and faecal sludge management will be piloted in a densely populated ward.
Description of good practices	The tool selected for raising awareness for hygiene and health issues and demand in the community is the **initial community meeting approach**. This tool is one of the activities in the *process ignition* step of the CLUES approach. (CLUES planning is a seven-step multi-sector and multiple-actor approach to urban sanitation planning.) The meeting includes fun and interactive elements to promote lively participation.
	The key components of the initial community meeting approach are as follows:
	1. Discussion of key environmental sanitation problems where a number of sanitation problems are listed with their suggested solutions. 2. A 'transect walk' (commonly used in CLTS). This approach helps community members see for themselves the status of latrines and dirty environments in the community and ignites collective community actions for improved latrines and their dirty environments. 3. Creating a map of the neighbourhood in a participatory mapping exercise (often referred to as community mapping). Mapping is a tool used to involve all community members in a practical and visual analysis of their sanitation situation. 4. Defining the project boundaries and area of intervention. In plenary, the community agrees upon the issues identified and states their willingness to tackle them. If they seem to be committed, the community leader representing the community as a whole signs a declaration form.

	5. A community taskforce is formed. This taskforce consists of committed and enthusiastic community members who are willing to be involved in the planning process by representing the interests and concerns of the community. The taskforce coordinates all hygiene and sanitation activities in the hamlet/village. They regularly follow-up with those households without improved latrines, carry out meetings with the community, and give feedback on progress to the street, government, and community.
Challenges	• Low-income communities are not always capable of self-financing the planning and implementation of improved environmental sanitation services. Advertisements at sanitation bazaar events, as well as radio jingles and brochures for toilet construction and improvements focus on microcredit products. • The taskforce lacks full support from the municipal implementation team, hamlet/street leader, and hamlet/street environment and sanitation committee. • Lack of follow-up on what has been planned and committed to by the community from the municipal implementation team to ensure that there are gradual improvements in toilet technologies, and to help sustain attitude changes. • The municipal implementation team fails to own and be committed to agreements, rules, and responsibilities.
Results	• 12 community sanitation action plans have been developed across the five wards. • Communities in the target areas have been sensitized and mobilized to a satisfactory level. In total, 2,991 community members participated in the community meetings, including 1,751 female and 1,240 male participants. • About 93% of neighbourhoods have been reached. • 52 community task forces have been formed. • A total of 52 initial community meetings were conducted in four wards of Iringa municipality: 11 in Kitwiru, 11 in Nduli, 13 in Kihesa, and 17 in Mtwivila. • Four community problems with regard to environmental sanitation were prioritized: poor latrine facilities or no latrine; poor drainage of waste water; poor management of solid waste; and poor water services. • Two environmental sanitation systems were identified (pour-flush toilet and Fossa Alterna). • Agreements were signed between target communities and Iringa municipal council for improvements to sanitation in their areas. • Project operation and maintenance regulations and procedures are currently being developed.
References	Lüthi, C., Morel, A., Tilley, E. and Ulrich, L. (2011) *Community-Led Urban Environmental Sanitation: CLUES. A Complete Guide for Decision Makers with 30 Tools*, Dübendorf, Switzerland, Eawag, UN Habitat, and WSSCC, http://www.eawag.ch/fileadmin/Domain1/Abteilungen/sandec/schwerpunkte/sesp/CLUES/CLUES_Guidelines.pdf [accessed 25 February 2018].

Case Study 8: IUWASH, Indonesia

Ika Francisca, USAID IUWASH PLUS Project, DAI, and Louis O'Brien, Chief of Party, USAID IUWASH PLUS Project, DAI

Context	Indonesia Urban Water, Sanitation and Hygiene (IUWASH) project was implemented in both formal and informal neighbourhoods in 54 large cities.
Implementing organization	USAID IUWASH.
Funding details	USAID provided US$39.6 million over five years. Note that funding for infrastructure was almost entirely leveraged from the Government of Indonesia (GOI) and other sources.
Objectives	An increase of 2,400,000 million people in urban areas with access to improved water supply.
	An increase of 250,000 people in urban areas with access to improved sanitation facilities.
	A decrease of 20% in the per unit water cost paid by the poor in targeted communities.
	100,000 people trained in WASH-related areas.
Dates	IUWASH ran from 2011 to 2016. A follow-on programme, IUWASH PLUS, started in 2016 and will run until 2021.
Sanitation solutions	Household septic systems, communal wastewater treatment plants (WWTPs), municipal-level septage treatment plants (STPs), and some sewerage systems.
Description of good practices	USAID IUWASH supported the adaptation of the GOI's *Sanitasi Total Berbaisis Masyarakat* (Community-Led Total Sanitation or STBM) programme for urban settings. IUWASH also sought to increase the capacity of water service providers, including *Perusahaan Daerah Air Minum* (local government-owned water utilities) and agencies providing sanitation services, notably by supporting the development of citywide sanitation strategies.
	The Indonesian Ministry of Health (MOH) has been very successful in implementing STBM in rural areas and embarking on an initiative to expand the programme to urban areas. Although various elements of STBM as it is implemented in rural areas could be applied in an urban setting (such as transect walks, triggering events, etc.), much needed to be adapted to the specific conditions confronted by urban dwellers, and especially the urban poor. This is because, unlike rural areas, household-level sanitation systems in urban centres are generally much more costly (as they must conform to more stringent regulations), and their longer-term operation and maintenance depend on much larger municipal-level systems (for safe septage collection, treatment, and disposal). In addition, urban communities can be less cohesive than those in rural areas and more difficult to organize due to the staggered schedules of urban residents (rendering traditional triggering approaches less effective). To assist in this process, USAID IUWASH worked in close contact with its GOI counterparts to develop an Urban Sanitation Promotion (USP) guide

to provide everyone involved in sector development with an overview of how municipal wastewater management systems operate, the required enabling environment that needs to be developed in urban sanitation, and their role in making this happen.

Building on the above, the MOH and USAID IUWASH conducted a series of three-day USP 'training of trainers' (TOT) programmes targeting local health personnel – and, in particular, sanitarians who are most closely involved in STBM implementation. Training covered the broad array of issues involved in USP – technical issues, regulatory concerns, finance, marketing, and communications – all of which are part of triggering households to invest in appropriate sanitation systems (toilets with proper septic tanks or connections to communal or citywide sewerage systems). At the end of the TOT, participants developed specific action plans to introduce urban-oriented STBM approaches to the community level. An important element of those plans related to the training and support of local health volunteers (*kaders*) in what has become known as 'multi-level sanitation marketing', which underscores the need for the engagement of many actors across the urban landscape.

Another key element involved the development of 'sanitation entrepreneurs' who can manage the construction of new sanitation systems, as well as the establishment of microfinance programmes to improve system affordability. The city of Probolinggo offers one example where, during a study tour to the neighbouring district of Jombang, about 20 STBM leaders (department heads, sanitarians, and others) met with that district's sanitation entrepreneurs to learn how they fund and operate their businesses and better understand how similar entrepreneurs could be developed in their city. Upon their return, a group of six new entrepreneurs was formed and further supported with a microfinance fund to aid low-income households in paying for their new systems. With the cost of new systems ranging from US$50 to US$200, weekly instalments are as low as US$1, quickly leading to 100 households obtaining new toilets with proper septic systems. Importantly, the city government of Probolinggo also intensified its own efforts to develop critical septage management systems.

Other examples include the district of Tangerang, where similar combined efforts in septage management planning, strong promotional programmes, and an important microfinance initiative to improve affordability led to more than 5,000 new household sanitation facilities being developed (reaching an estimated 25,000 people). A similar programme in the district of Bandung also resulted in 1,500 new proper yet affordable toilets with septic tanks being put in place. Under another initiative involving multiple cities and districts, it is estimated that close to 200,000 people were connected to communal sanitation systems that had previously been underutilized due to a lack of promotional programming.

The programme's work also extended to promoting household connections to large-scale sewerage systems and communal-level WWTPs. Although scores of such systems had been constructed, many were severely under-subscribed as households were reluctant to connect. Their reluctance was due to several reasons, often revolving around both the cost of connecting and perceived shortcomings of such systems (including frequent clogging of pipes, related odours, etc.). In response, IUWASH worked to improve promotional programming and triggering activities, but ensured that these were supplemented with customer education programmes regarding system use (for example, on what can and cannot be disposed of through the systems) and substantial work in strengthening local institutions that could take responsibility for long-term technical oversight and support (to respond to customer complaints in the case of large-scale sewerage systems or provide technical support to the CBOs charged with managing communal WWTPs).

All of the above was supported by a wide range of promotional and informational materials, including brochures, posters, videos, small plastic models of septic systems, etc. At the household level, messaging was also expanded beyond the idea that sanitation improvements are important for health, appealing to people's often stronger desire for increased convenience, status, and sense of security that improved sanitation facilities can provide.

These efforts are now continuing under the USAID IUWASH PLUS programme, which is strongly aligned with water and sanitation SDGs. In the realm of urban sanitation, it is seeking to move 250,000 low-income people classified as practising OD to the status of having access to 'improved sanitation'; and another 250,000 from their current level of access to 'safely managed sanitation' status.

The broad strategy that guides the IUWASH PLUS programme's sanitation work calls for strong collaboration with national GOI agencies and for the provision of significant assistance to local government partners. The latter includes assisting local government institutions in: engaging with low-income communities to develop long-term solutions to their WASH needs; developing municipal wastewater management institutional capacity to meet SDG requirements; and facilitating required infrastructure improvement from household to municipal levels. This has been supplemented by IUWASH PLUS work in developing wealth determination methodologies; behaviour change formative research and strategy development; marketing research; spatial analysis programming; budget advocacy and policy development; the establishment of WASH microfinance programmes; and technical support related to septage management planning, from household septic systems to municipal WWTPs. Further information on the above and other USAID IUWASH PLUS programming is available at https://www.iuwashplus.or.id/.

Lessons
- Work on sanitation in an urban setting is substantially different from work in rural areas, requiring approaches that go far beyond triggering and embrace a much broader enabling environment.
- Stakeholder consultation and involvement are critical to the development of solutions that local partners can sustain and build upon.
- Urban sanitation requires the development of a robust enabling environment to address important promotional, institutional, and technical issues. These all require ongoing attention.
- Planning sanitation interventions in urban settings needs to account not only for the number and type of toilets, but also for the availability of desludging services, planned development of off-site systems, the socioeconomic profile of targeted communities, ownership, and the availability of microfinance and trained SMEs in the area.
- Community exchange visits are a powerful tool for engaging and triggering other communities into action.

Results	- 2,246,005 people obtained access to safe water supplies.
- 256,055 people have gained access to improved sanitation facilities.
- 89,566 people (33% of whom are women) have benefited from project training activities.
- 239 government institutions and civil society organizations (CSOs) implement WatSan programmes.
- 47 local governments increased local budget allocation and improved their policies to support improvement in the WatSan sector.
- Five local government wastewater management units were established and operational.
References	USAID and IUWASH (n.d.a) *Optimizing Coverage of Existing Master Meter and Triggering Community-based Total Sanitation in Sidoarjo District, East Java Province*, information sheet, USAID and Indonesia Urban Water, Sanitation, and Hygiene (IUWASH), https://www.iuwashplus.or.id/cms/wp-content/uploads/2017/04/Info-Sheet-Grants-in-Lemah-Putro-EN.pdf [accessed 25 February 2018].
USAID and IUWASH (n.d.b) *Program Profile: Community-based Total Sanitation Approach in Probolinggo City*, USAID and Indonesia Urban Water, Sanitation, and Hygiene (IUWASH), Surabaya, https://www.iuwashplus.or.id/cms/wp-content/uploads/2017/05/Program-Profile-STBM-in-Probolinggo-EN.pdf [accessed 25 February 2018].
IUWASH (2015) *Improving Lifestyle and Health: A Guide to Urban Sanitation Promotion*, IUWASH, Jakarta, https://www.iuwashplus.or.id/cms/wp-content/uploads/2017/04/Guide-to-Urban-Sanitation-Promotion-EN.pdf [accessed 23 March 2018].

Case Study 9: Kabwe, Zambia

Wiscot Mathews Mwanza, Plan Zambia

Context	Nakoli is an informal neighbourhood of 2,200 households located in a flood-prone area. Katonda is a planned township of approximately 26,000 households. Both are part of Kabwe, a provincial town in Kabwe Central Province, Zambia.
Implementing organizations	WASTE Netherlands with Plan International Zambia.
Funding details	Funded by the Dutch Ministry of Foreign Affairs and SNS Reaal.
Objectives	Water and Sewerage Utility Kabwe, in collaboration with small- and medium-sized local entrepreneurs, to provide sustainable sanitation services to poor peri-urban communities.
Dates	Ended in 2015 but as of February 2018 is being considered for another 18 months.
Sanitation solution	Urine diversion dry toilets.
Description of good practices	• The approach included CLTS, sanitation marketing, government enforcement, and demand creation combined with capacity building for group savings and loans organizations and community-based entrepreneurs. • Demand creation included triggering designed to highlight the contamination of wells from unimproved toilets. For example, households were given water-testing kits to test water sources themselves for faecal contamination. Teams visited the next day and households were asked to present the results to community meetings. • There was the start of public–private partnerships (PPPs) between community-based enterprises (constructors, transporters, and farmers) and the local government (Kabwe municipal council) based on the concepts of sustainable sanitation and closing the loop (reuse). • An initial agreement was made with the Zambian National Building Society for sanitation loans. However, the application process took too long. WASTE then worked with a local microfinance institution, the Community Empowerment Fund (CEF). The CEF does not give loans in cash but in materials and labour. A bill of quantity is filled out listing all the materials needed for construction – households can then reduce loans if they can source materials in other ways. Community-based entrepreneurs then have 30 days to complete the toilets. • CLTS triggering was just one component of a larger behaviour change communication strategy which included door-to-door campaigns, community radio shows and public address systems, posters in local languages, and using church leaders to promote sanitation messages. • The community was also brought together – across all four blocks – at a toilet design meeting where three different designs were discussed and the community used pair ranking to decide which one they wanted. Urine diversion dry toilets (UDDTs) came out on top and it was these that were promoted and monitored – they were also endorsed by local government.

Challenges	• The problems in Kabwe were OD, flying toilets, and the contamination of drinking water wells by traditional pit latrines – triggering tools were designed around this. • The idea of using CLTS triggering to create demand was something that came later and consequently there was no funding for training and development of community champions. • The application process for loans was initially tiresome and loans were significantly delayed as they had to be signed off by a board based in Lusaka – WASTE later established a partnership with the CEF (see above). • The idea of sustainable sanitation and the reuse of excreta was not supported by Kabwe municipal council officials in the engineering and public health departments because they lacked the expertise to judge what is actually needed to implement the proposed service delivery system and to develop new by-laws and revenue systems that should facilitate these interventions in peri-urban areas.
Lessons	• The concept of a sustainable sanitation chain consisting of a service component and a value chain is not feasible if important conditions are not met. These include awareness and change of behaviour, economies of density, a certain level of income, infrastructure, and enforcement of regulations to pay fees for waste collection. • Success is reliant on a number of different stakeholders that often move at different paces, increasing the number of bottlenecks. In Kabwe, working with the CEF rather than Zambia National Building Society meant that loans could be processed faster and designing the right financial product became more feasible. • A mass campaign to raise awareness in peri-urban areas is not a good substitute for CLTS. Large and populous settlements need a different strategy to mobilize people, to change their behaviour, and to make changes sustainable. Local cadres such as environmental health technicians (EHTs), neighbourhood health committees, their voluntary staff, and councillors are the first and most strategic target group. • Application of this approach in peri-urban areas requires the availability of an experienced facilitator or coordinator who knows its pitfalls and problems.
References	Myers, J. (2016) *Plan Netherlands' Experience of Using a CLTS Approach in Urban Environments*, Plan Nederland, Amsterdam, www.communityledtotalsanitation.org/sites/communityledtotalsanitation.org/files/Urban_CLTS_Plan.pdf [accessed 5 September 2016].

Case Study 10: Logo, Nigeria

Nanpet Chuktu, Programme Manager, RUSHPIN, United Purpose, and Shadrack Guusu, LGA Technical Support Officer, RUSHPIN, United Purpose

Context	CLTS was used in four peri-urban, low-density small towns in Logo LGA (local government area), Benue State, Nigeria.
Implementing organization	United Purpose is the executing agency implementing the Rural Sanitation and Hygiene Promotion Programme in Nigeria (RUSHPIN).
Funding details	RUSHPIN is supported by the Global Sanitation Fund, a pooled global fund established by the Water Supply and Sanitation Collaborative Council (WSSCC). In Mdadyul (457 households), US$6,154 was spent; in Abeda (1,025 households), US$3,846 was spent. Both costs included five verification visits.
Objectives	• To achieve increased improved sanitation coverage and hygiene behaviours through a demand-led process, empowering local communities to improve their sanitation and hygiene practices. • To strengthen political commitment to increase resources for sanitation and hygiene.
Dates	Ongoing.
Sanitation solutions	Anything that is fly-proof and separates faeces from human contact.
Description of good practices/challenges	Mob triggering is a CLTS approach used in two small towns in peri-urban and urban centres which maximizes the shock effect of the triggering process by engaging the entire urban centre, with people meeting in different clusters at the same time. In Anyiin town in Logo LGA (Benue State), a peri-urban town of 11,517, and Sankwala town in Obanliku LGA (Cross River State), a town with a population of 5,429 people, tools similar to the traditional CLTS triggering approach were used followed shortly by follow-up visits. A single team moved day by day, engaging clusters of between 35 and 50 households in the triggering process. The team of facilitators observed that by the second or third day, clusters were registering very few people attending the triggering sessions. There was a loss of the shock effect of shame and disgust among the people gathered at the triggering sessions. People knew what was going to happen next during the sessions. People from other clusters had either heard from their friends what the triggering sessions were all about, or had witnessed the triggering sessions the day before. The result was a long, slow process to becoming ODF for the individual clusters in the urban centre. It took an average of six months for each cluster to become ODF. Action plans were weak. Cluster heads were either not present at sessions or did not feel a sense of collective action towards behaviour change. Mbadyul is a peri-urban town of 457 households and an estimated population of 3,634, while Abeda town, in Logo LGA (Benue State), has 1,025 households with a population of 4,506 people. Ten triggering teams of six CLTS facilitators each were established, and each team triggered and engaged clusters in Mbadyul at the same time.

The effect of this was that more than half the small town was engaged on the same day at around the same time in the CLTS triggering event, while in Abeda the entire town was engaged at the same time using 16 CLTS triggering teams. Action points were agreed upon and became a source of competition, with clusters competing to be the first to become ODF. Some key steps taken by the team of CLTS facilitators are listed below:

- Triggering teams are established to match the number of communities within the settlement. CLTS facilitators are drawn from the local government WASH unit, CSO partners, and community volunteer groups that emerge in the course of programme implementation.
- All CLTS communities within each settlement are mobilized for triggering at the same time.
- Each triggering team is allocated one CLTS community within the settlement and all triggering sessions are carried out simultaneously.

To ensure that a good percentage of the population attend and participate in the triggering, the following steps are taken to minimize distraction:

- A work-free day (Saturday) was selected for triggering.
- The triggering day was strategically picked to coincide with the town's monthly environmental sanitation day, when no forms of commercial activity or movement are allowed before 9 a.m.

Results 1,482 households from Mbadyul and Abeda constructed and use latrines and both are now ODF. It took six to eight weeks for these two settlements to become ODF.

Lessons
- Target the rural clusters around the town first and support them to become ODF. This builds the confidence and competence of the local triggering teams that will later reach out to the urban areas.
- Selecting a suitable day for most individuals to be present and at home is key to ensuring that no one is left behind.
- Using Natural Leaders from neighbouring communities in post-triggering activities is effective.
- Engaging many clusters at the same time allows for maximum shock effect.

References Guusu, S. and Chuktu, N. (n.d.) *Mob Triggering: An Urban CLTS Approach to Reaching Whole Clusters. The Experience of GSF-supported RUSHPIN Programme, Logo LGA, Benue State, Nigeria*, United Purpose, unpublished report.

Case Study 11: Mathare 10, Nairobi, Kenya

Samuel Musembi Musyoki, Country Director, Plan International Zambia, formerly Strategic Director of Programmes, Plan International Kenya, and Rose Nyawira, co-founder of Top Notch Empowerment Centre, previously Project Officer, Plan International Kenya

Context	Mathare 10 is made up of four densely populated informal neighbourhoods – Nyangau, Thayu, Mabtini, and Mashimoni – with a population of 20,000. It is part of Mathare, the second largest informal settlement in Kenya. With an estimated population of over 200,000 inhabitants, it covers an area of about 5 square kilometres.
	The land is privately owned and housing is a mix of permanent and temporary dwellings which are mostly made of mud and tin and lack sanitation facilities; tenants are forced to use flying toilets. Raw sewerage openly drains in from the nearby suburbs and into the nearby Nairobi River.
Implementing organizations	Plan International Kenya, Community Cleaning Services (CCS), and the County Government of Nairobi.
Funding details	The project was co-financed by the Dutch Ministry of Foreign Affairs and Plan Netherland with a budget of €35,000.
Objectives	• Ensure that adequate sanitation and hygiene practices are used by all. • Empower communities to develop their own sanitation and hygiene services as well as maintain them. • Develop a U-CLTS model and share lessons for scaling-up. • Establish a cooperation network between research and civil society institutions for U-CLTS and CLTS. • Get local entrepreneurs active in helping households climb the sanitation ladder.
Dates	Project ended in 2014.
Sanitation solutions	• Triggering residents to use and improve existing facilities. • Building toilets for housing blocks and public facilities using funds from landlords and private entrepreneurs. • Use of pay-per-use toilets. • Piloting 'Freshlife' toilets, where biogas is produced and used for commercial cooking and boiling water for bathing. • A sewer line was built as part of a slum-upgrading initiative.
Description of good practices	• Obtaining buy-in and establishing a core team (CCS, Plan International, local administration, and County Government of Nairobi) to mobilize communities and provide leadership in the U-CLTS process. • Capacity development through hands-on U-CLTS training of 30 selected community leaders, youth, and government public health officers based in Mathare ward. Working with youth to enhance community sanitation profile data and information through participatory GIS mapping, participatory video, and social media to tell the story behind the maps and the data. • Community and targeted triggering (schools, business premises, churches, and landlords) using participatory tools (mapping,

transect walk, faecal flow charts, shit calculations, and ignition moments), leading to the development of a community sanitation profile and action plans.
- Presenting data and information with the view of providing evidence to influence policymakers and service providers. Using the data with young entrepreneurs to initiate and grow their own businesses providing sanitation services, predominantly toilet cleaning, garbage collection, and light maintenance of sanitation facilities. Mathare Natural Leaders and U-CLTS facilitators using the maps and data to hold round-table engagements with targeted stakeholders and service providers, including the City Council of Nairobi and the private sector. Using information collected during the U-CLTS process to conduct targeted triggering for institutions – the City Council Planning, City Cleansing, and Community Development Departments, the Ministry of Public Health and Sanitation, international NGOs, private-sector sanitation entrepreneurs, academic and research institutions, and the international community.
- Bringing together Natural Leaders, landlords, civic leaders, and government institutions to find solutions to problems such as the limited space for building sanitation facilities.
- Bringing together human rights advocacy groups with research and academic institutions to provide an opportunity to gather evidence to influence the city's Planning Department.
- Sustained engagement with media to reinforce key messages of ending OD and influence policymakers and service providers. The project partnered with Kenya Broadcasting Cooperation and used the popular comedy show Vitimbi, which Natural Leaders drew on to start community conversations challenging poor hygiene practices. Also establishing the Mathare Valley blog: https://matharevalley.wordpress.com/category/sanitation/. The blog attracted responses and support from different stakeholders, including the media, NGOs, the UN, and donors.
- Identifying Natural Leaders and champions within the community, landlords, civic leaders, provincial administration, government institutions, and NGOs.

Challenges

- Participation during triggering was low as people are busy during the day.
- A transient population resulting in a low sense of community cohesion. Most people living in Mathare, as in other informal settlements, will only stay until they find somewhere more appropriate to live.
- Limited or no space for mapping on the ground as streets are very narrow, busy, and dirty.
- Land tenure issues increase insecurity for investment in private sanitation facilities.
- Limited space for the construction of sanitation facilities.
- Lack of political will, coupled with politicization of sanitation services. U-CLTS is seen as both a threat and an opportunity to the vested interests of different groups and powerful actors.
- Weak coordination, regulation, and enforcement of tenancy and sanitation city by-laws and standards or types of technology to be used.
- Poor sludge management practices – there are no organized services to manage sludge after pit emptying.

Results	• Increased demand and collective action to engage with the duty bearers and urban sanitation service providers.
• A significant reduction in OD and flying toilets. OD areas were cleaned up and used as play areas for children, open markets for small-scale traders, and vegetable gardens. Hanging toilets were also demolished.
• Increase in the number of toilets constructed by landlords and private entrepreneurs.
• Demand for mobile cleaning teams increased, including from churches, schools, restaurants, etc.
• Local administration used the U-CLTS outcome for effective mobilization of the community and enforcement of by-laws to ensure that landlords constructed sanitation facilities for the tenants.
• Acceptance by Nairobi City County key departments of U-CLTS as a methodology for doing sanitation work. An increased demand for U-CLTS – 40 more facilitators have been trained and are working in six other informal settlements in Nairobi. In addition, the uptake and scale-up of U-CLTS by more organizations working in other informal settlements in Nairobi and in other counties, including Nakuru (see Case Study 12), Kisumu, and Trukana.
• Development of Natural Leaders (mostly women and youth) who are now spearheading strong CBOs that have put sanitation and community empowerment on the political agenda.
• Mathare 10 has been the focus of several national and international learning visits.
• The formation of the Nairobi Environmental Sanitation and Hygiene movement was a key achievement. The movement has ensured that sanitation remains at the top of the agenda in any development, not just in Mathare but in all informal settlements in Nairobi. It even influenced the 2017 Nairobi county environmental management policy, which now includes community groups in the collection and management of waste at the community level (in informal settlements).
Lessons	• Proper coordination and the setting of clear roles and responsibilities for the different actors involved in U-CLTS are important in helping to avoid conflict and duplication of efforts.
• CLTS was a very effective tool in mobilizing and galvanizing tenants or communities to demand their right to sanitation from the duty bearers.
• The cash economy in urban areas creates opportunities for investment in sanitation as a business – most people would pay to access better sanitation facilities.
• Visits by government officials and influential stakeholders along with activation sessions and subsequent activities encouraged the community to change their sanitation practices.
• Given the transient nature and mobility of the community, it is important to agree with the local leadership on the most suitable time for triggering.
• The lack of safety for women and girls using communal toilets was an issue that drove them to demand household-level sanitation facilities from the landlords.
• While enthusiasm to end OD was high, there was a genuine lack of space to put up sanitation facilities, which meant that hard negotiation was needed with landlords to convert some of the rental rooms to toilets.

- Precarious land tenure was a major hindrance for entrepreneurs looking to invest in sanitation.
- The use of GIS and social media helps systematize U-CLTS data and present it in a more powerful way – appealing to policymakers and decision-makers.
- In Kenya, household visits by local leaders as well as government officials proved successful at encouraging households to participate.

References

Musyoki, S. (2010) *Piloting CLTS in an Urban Setting: Diary of Progress in Mathare 10, Nairobi, Kenya*, http://www.communityledtotalsanitation.org/sites/communityledtotalsanitation.org/files/media/Mathare_blog_all.pdf [accessed 7 November 2017].

Quayle, T. (2012) 'UCLTS in Mathare 10, Nairobi', ACCESSanitation case study, http://www.communityledtotalsanitation.org/resource/access-case-study-uclts-mathare-10-nairobi [accessed 25 February 2018].

Case Study 12: Nakuru, Kenya

Peter Murigi, WASH Technical Officer at ACTED, formerly Urban WASH Specialist at Practical Action, and Lucy Stevens, Senior Policy and Practice Adviser, Practical Action

Context	The Realising the Right to Total Sanitation project in Nakuru low-income settlement targets two informal settlements in Kenya's fourth largest city, with a population of 308,000 (according to the 2009 census). The informal settlements were Rhonda (approximately 22,000 households) and Kaptembwo (approximately 25,500 households).
Implementing organizations	Practical Action and Umande Trust.
Funding details	£728,000 over 39 months (three years plus a three-month inception phase) from Comic Relief.
Objectives	• Engage 95% of residents across two settlements in the CLTS process and identify and agree sanitation needs for their areas. • By the end of the project, have no OD or flying toilets in four out of six zones in the settlements. • 60% of residents to have access to adequate on-plot sanitation and at-point handwashing facilities and the communities to have the organizational capacity and finance to complete the remaining 40% after the project ends. • U-CLTS scaled-up beyond the project area. • Minimum of 20 pit emptiers working with the Municipal Council of Nakuru (MCN) and Nakuru Water and Sanitation Services Company, ensuring that services maintain better hygiene conditions and comply with sanitation regulations. • Train at least 100 artisans in constructing toilets that meet standards agreed through the project and using new technologies. • MCN initiates CLTS in another slum with the support of Umande Trust independently of the project.
Dates	January 2012–March 2015.
Sanitation solutions	• Pit latrines (27%); • Ventilated improved pit (VIP) latrines (53%); • Pour-flush toilets with septic tank (20%); • 1 'bio-centre' community sanitation facility.
Description of good practices	• Participatory GIS was used to map sanitation facilities and their current conditions, to identify OD hotspots and to understand the scale of the challenge. • The capacity of public health officers and Community Health Volunteers was strengthened on CLTS approaches and the adoption of low-cost sanitation technologies such as gulper technology. • Tenants, landlords, financial institutions, pit emptiers, waste pickers, schools, and artisans were engaged in CLTS in order to tackle the issue of sanitation improvement.

- Partnership with the Ministry of Health helped ensure scale-up and sustainability. National government and county government were engaged to ensure that policies, guidelines, standards, and by-laws exist and are enforced to direct urban CLTS processes and targets. These need to be stringent enough to ensure that solutions are safe and sustainable in the urban context (considering the full sanitation chain) while also being pro-poor. Practical Action's work in Nakuru highlighted the need to negotiate these with authorities to ensure that standards are realistic and achievable by local communities.
- Participatory technology development approaches were used to develop appropriate, low-cost sanitation facilities, with a set of designs approved and available 'off the shelf' from the county government.
- A referral letter was issued to landlords to acquire approved sanitation technologies or designs from the Department of Planning, Nakuru county government, for sanitation improvement, reducing the cost of constructing these designs.
- Landlords were supported in identifying trained artisans to engage in the construction of appropriate low-cost sanitation technologies.
- Council officers and community members had an exposure visit to Mathare 10 in Nairobi (see Case Study 11).
- Visual toolkits and hygiene promotional tools were developed.
- Access to finance was made easier through an arrangement with K-Rep Bank (now Sidian Bank), although most of the landlords mobilized their own resources to invest.
- The project reached out to informal-sector workers (pit emptiers) who formed an association that gave them a voice and recognition. The county government recognized the value of their work, but also the need to improve quality and safety.

Challenges
- It was difficult to achieve requirements for at-point handwashing facilities.
- Absentee landlords (around 30%) were the hardest to reach.
- Despite making finance available, most landlords opted to use their own resources. Securing sufficient resources can delay construction work.
- The existence of subsidy-based sanitation programmes in other parts of Nakuru slightly affected the project as some landlords failed to construct latrines as they were waiting for the subsidy programme to support them.
- Waste pickers stole the handwashing facilities, and soap was also stolen. This was mitigated by the use of bowls within their personal rooms and by the provision of concrete handwashing facilities adjacent to the toilet.
- No ongoing budget for travel and materials is available to public health officers to continue to scale up the approach.

Results
- 135,431 people were engaged in the CLTS process.
- There are ODF areas in four out of six zones in the two informal settlements, although these have not been officially declared due to regulations around the location of handwashing stations.
- Through the CLTS-based approach, 140 community mobilizers and 15 Department of Health public health officers were trained and they continued to support scaling-up of CLTS in the project area and beyond.

	- Nakuru county government Department of Health adopted a CLTS approach and managed to trigger 10 more villages during the project period. Currently, they are using a CLTS approach countywide. - 1,603 new safe and adequate on-plot sanitation structures were constructed, providing security, privacy, and dignity to users, and which are safe for use by women, the elderly, and children, and 601 existing structures were renovated, benefiting 58,260 residents. - By the end of the project, 95% of residents and schoolchildren were aware of and had adopted good hygiene and handwashing practices (68,879 people), with a widespread sense of individual responsibility for maintaining the sanitary environment, and 60% of households had simple handwashing facilities in their homes. - 28 pit emptiers came together to form an association, legitimizing their work. - At least 100 artisans were trained and employed in constructing toilets that meet standards agreed through the project and are using new technologies. During the project period, 37 pit emptiers and 109 construction artisans were trained and engaged in FSM and construction works to ensure that sanitation facilities are improved.
Lessons	- MCN has fully adopted the CLTS approach in informal settlements in Nakuru. - The Realising the Right to Total Sanitation project in Nakuru low-income settlement represented a very important example of urban application and adaptation of CLTS methodology. - The project provided an excellent example of good partnership working with key stakeholder institutions (Nakuru County Department of Health, Planning and Environment, and Nakuru Water and Sanitation Services Company (NAWASSCO)), leading to wider replication, influence on policy, and good opportunities for impact at scale. Continued sharing of experiences and lessons learned will help guide county and national levels in developing the U-CLTS protocol for the verification and certification of urban areas as ODF. - The project team has built strong and lasting relationships with the Ministry of Health and NAWASSCO that will facilitate future engagement of manual pit emptiers in filling the gap in the FSM process. - The promotion of other technologies by other partners and stakeholders within the project areas will help in filling the gaps in the sanitation value chain. - Many landlords invested in improved sanitation facilities using their own resources. - Communities responded fast once triggered and landlords were brought on board and linked to credit arrangements and the availability of artisans.
References	Hueso, A. (2013) 'Sanitation in Nakuru's low-income urban areas', CLTS blog, http://www.communityledtotalsanitation.org/blog/sanitation-nakuru-s-low-income-urban-areas [accessed 25 February 2018].

Pasteur, K. and Prabhakaran, P. (2015) *Lessons in Urban Community-Led Total Sanitation from Nakuru, Kenya*, Rugby, Practical Action, www.communityledtotalsanitation.org/sites/communityledtotalsanitation.org/files/PracticalAction_LessonsOnUrbanCLTSNakuruKenya_Apr2015.pdf [accessed 7 October 2017].

Practical Action (n.d.b) *Total Sanitation in Nakuru Slums*, collation of project materials, video, blogs, papers, etc., Rugby, Practical Action, https://practicalaction.org/realising-the-right-to-total-sanitation-in-nakuru-slums [accessed 25 February 2018].

Stevens, L. (2013) 'Realising the right to total sanitation: hybrid Community-Led Total Sanitation in Nakuru, Kenya', Practical Action blog, https://practicalaction.org/blog/where-we-work/kenya/realising-the-right-to-total-sanitation-hybrid-clts-in-nakuru/ [accessed 25 February 2018].

Case Study 13: New Delhi, India

Brendon Dhu and Biswajeet Mukherjee, Manager, Feedback Foundation

Context	Nalla, Delit Eckta, Arjun, and Bandu settlements, New Delhi.
Implementing organization	Feedback Foundation.
Description of good practices	• *Pocket triggering*. This is effective in tackling situations where community-wide triggering attempts have not reached enough people in a community. Local leaders and emerging champions are encouraged to arrange triggering and take a bigger role in triggering exercises. The outcome is clusters where people have increased motivation and awareness; these clusters then begin to merge and form a complete network of awareness and collective action throughout a settlement. • *Morning follow-up*. U-CLTS triggering normally leads to the formation of a community vigilance committee. The vigilance committee visits households at around 5 a.m. daily to support the committee and emerging Natural Leaders. This has three outcomes: 1) defective or unused toilets become active and used again; 2) all people with a household toilet will stop OD; and 3) people start to understand that the problem is collective and requires a collective solution and therefore people with toilets will begin to shun the practice of OD and actively seek to influence those continuing to OD by finding solutions such as the temporary sharing of toilets. • *Household-level follow-up*. Field staff follow up with households to discuss the personal sanitation situation of each household and encourage household members to get involved in the community-wide movement. Initially, household follow-up focuses on those already with toilets. Once those who have toilets come to understand that they are not protected unless the whole community stops OD they become more concerned and active. These people set an example, and in some cases offer their toilets to neighbours as a temporary solution. Household meetings may include some small triggering activities such as the calculation of the medical costs of diarrhoea-related illness and discussions about toilet technologies and budgets.
Results	• Where community-wide triggering participation is low, targeted pocket triggering helped influence a wider range of groups within a community. • Leach pit latrines were the best onsite technology option for Delhi's sandy soils. Leach pits help reduce the challenge and cost of dealing with the safe removal of sludge when compared with septic tanks.
Lessons	• Redefining triggering to better suit the complexities of urban contexts may include less focus on triggering events that involve the whole community and more on pocket triggering for the specific needs of various groups within a community. Using existing and emerging community CLTS champions can help improve understanding and the effectiveness of pocket triggering, and advocate for collective sanitation improvements in their community.

- Household follow-up and personalized triggering are useful for engaging parts of the community with limited exposure to previous community-wide campaigns to stop OD. Support by CLTS facilitation staff for the morning follow-up visits by the vigilance committee is an important tool in challenging urban contexts. When leadership is weak or community champions lack legitimacy, external support at the morning follow-up visits can consolidate community-wide effort. However, only people from within the community can take a role in shaming open defecators.
- Diverse and innovative methods to announce triggering meetings are used, including parades through the lanes, roving theatre and musical performances, and the use of influential celebrities and local religious groups. Further research and documentation of experiences is suggested.
- U-CLTS should focus on identifying and building social capital as part of a longer pre-triggering process.
- Collaboration with government and service providers from the outset is vital.
- Lack of space for toilet construction was a common problem. Household follow-up can help to enable collective solutions around labour, land tenure, or finance that bring the challenge back to the community scale.
- Community toilets are a valuable part of the total sanitation solution. U-CLTS helped the community collaborate on improved operation and maintenance of toilets, and to demand government support for repairs and upgrades.

References

- Dhu, B. (n.d.) *Challenges and Innovations of Urban Community-Led Total Sanitation: Case Study Findings from New Delhi, India*, unpublished report.

Case Study 14: Ribaué and Rapale, Mozambique

Alfonso Alvestegui, Senior Water and Sanitation Specialist, World Bank Group, formerly Urban Towns WASH Programme Manager, UNICEF Mozambique, and Ann Thomas, Sanitation and Hygiene Adviser, Eastern and Southern Africa, UNICEF

Context	The Small Towns WASH Programme in Nampula Province, Mozambique included using CLTS techniques in parts of Ribaué (population 26,000) and Rapale (19,000). Both are low-density peri-urban small rural towns (small district hubs). It was found that OD rates were high on the outer edges of the towns. Both towns demonstrated potential for high economic and population growth.
Implementing organization	UNICEF.
Funding details	AusAID.
Objectives	To increase access to safe water and effective sanitation services and to improve hygiene knowledge and practices. This would be delivered through: • improving household and public infrastructure and behaviours; • developing Sanitation Master Plans; and • improving school sanitation and water supply.
Dates	2012–14.
Sanitation solutions	• Pit latrines • Public latrines (in markets and schools)
Description of good practices	• It should be recognized that small towns contain a mix of housing and infrastructure: from very urban, grid-like, densely packed housing to very rural, large plots with livestock and scattered housing as one nears the periphery. Consequently, a uniform programming approach is not always desirable nor practical, particularly as behaviours also tend to reflect a rural–urban continuum. • A useful framework for analysis is to consider sanitation at three levels: household, collection, and final treatment. This could allow for in-situ upgrading and treatment and/or onsite facilities coupled with sludge collection and final treatment, condominial sewerage systems or central sewerage. The availability of piped water or wastewater production will be a factor in determining the feasibility of the various collection and treatment options.

		Infrastructure needed	Interventions	Financial responsibility for infrastructure
	Household	Safely managed sanitation depends on context. Can include: • improved pit latrines • septic tanks that can be emptied	• CLTS • Technical support via government and partners • Sanitation marketing • Block competitions	Household – latrine and pit upgrading

	Infrastructure needed	Interventions	Financial responsibility for infrastructure
Collection	• Pit emptying service • Sewerage connections and mains installed	• Training of pit emptiers • Purchase of *vacutugs* (small vacuum tankers) • Sanitation marketing • Regulation and enforcement of pit designs • Sewerage tariff and cost-recovery plan	Municipality
Final treatment	FSM		Municipality

- CLTS was used in the rural areas of the towns, which still practised OD, while Participatory Hygiene and Sanitation Transformation (PHAST) was used in the more urban areas to promote the upgrading of sanitation facilities. Interpersonal communication during the CLTS process helped maintain momentum for households to move up the sanitation ladder.
- Mixed-media communication techniques were used, such as radios and mobile units to record and broadcast video. The community radio sessions included children and local leaders and provided a platform for debate on sanitation and hygiene.
- A sanitation competition between *barrios* (neighbourhoods) in Mozambique challenged block leaders to mobilize their blocks to have the highest levels of improved latrines.
- A sanitation champion was elected within the municipal sanitation working group and tasked primarily with advocating for funding and prioritization of the Sanitation Master Plan and also with oversight of the plan.

Results

By the end of 2014:
- Over 14,000 households had onsite sanitation.
- 16,050 people had new handwashing facilities.
- The public sanitation facilities had a capacity for 1,730 people, including 575 people with disabilities.
- Solid waste collection and disposal services had been strengthened.
- Sanitation Master Plans had been developed to provide guidance and support in outlining options for development and increased capacity of the local supply sector and government to support sanitation in these districts, both rural and urban.

Lessons

- The lack of homogeneity, the disbursement of the population, difficulties in congregating the community, and differences in behaviours (OD versus upgrading) made it necessary to supplement traditional community mobilization techniques with broader communication and a demand-generation campaign.

- The design of sanitation programmes in small towns has to be flexible and context-specific. The programme started with an initial set of proposed actions or a 'basic package'. This evolved based on: the specific characteristics of small towns; baseline results; Sanitation Master Plans; surveys of people's willingness to pay; and analysis of barriers to improved sanitation.
- Small towns' sanitation programmes should include an institutional sanitation component, as interventions in health centres, schools, and marketplaces will have a significant impact on health and sanitation conditions in both the towns and the whole district, including rural areas.
- Menstrual hygiene management and school sanitation in particular can be powerful entry points for low-income community engagement and mobilization.
- Developing sanitation markets in small towns is an opportunity to tap into rural markets that rely on those towns (i.e. district centres) for markets and other consumer goods. This experience demonstrated that rural communities would use and benefit from sanitation services available in small towns.
- Not all entrepreneurs are good sanitation service providers and the sanitation business does not generate enough revenue for a stand-alone business. There are masons and artisans in small towns who are willing to become sanitation entrepreneurs but there are clear success factors for promoting sanitation services. For Mozambique, these included selecting people who already have experience as masons, are already engaged in the home construction industry, and have good local contacts.
- Rural sanitation mobilization tools are applicable in the small town context but may need to be supplemented with other demand-generation approaches, as was the case in Mozambique. This would help ensure the saturation of messages and the ability to differentially target populations in a community with varying baseline behaviours.
- A broad range of sanitation options should be considered in water supply feasibility studies.
- Capacity building for local government and utilities should support the long-term planning and costing of sanitation infrastructure.

References

Thomas, A. and Alvestegui, A. (2015) 'Sanitation in small towns: experience from Mozambique', Eastern and Southern Africa Learning Series, Nairobi, UNICEF, www.unicef.org/esaro/WASH-Field-Small-Towns-low-res.pdf [accessed 9 November 2017].

Muller, M. and Beaver, K. (2013) Water Supply, Sanitation and Hygiene in Nampula Province (NAMWASH), Mozambique, Evaluation Report, Water and Development Management and Ipsos MORI, https://dfat.gov.au/about-us/publications/Documents/mozambique-namwash-evaluation-2013.pdf [accessed 25 February 2018].

Government of Mozambique, Australian Aid, and UNICEF (2014) NAMWASH Programme: Phase 1 Progress Report, January–December 2013, unpublished report.

Case Study 15: Small towns in Northern and Southern Nigeria

Kabiru O. Abass, Department of Cooperative Economics and Management, Nnamdi Azikiwe University, Chinyere Umuoche, Small Town Water and Sanitation Agency, and Professor Charles Onugu, Centre for Community and Rural Development, Nnamdi Azikiwe University

Context	The project was implemented in low/peri-urban small- and medium-sized towns and some informal neighbourhoods/slum fishing communities in Yobe State, Northern Nigeria, and Anambra and Cross River States, Southern Nigeria.
Implementing organizations	Ministry of Water Resources and a combination of government agencies and NGOs in Yobe, Anambra, and Cross River States.
Funding details	Funded by the European Union, state government, local governments, and communities.
Objectives	• Reduce the incidence of water-related diseases. • Build sustainable structures and sustain ODF and total sanitation. • Strengthen policies, laws, and the capacity of water and sanitation institutions.
Dates	Ended in 2017.
Sanitation solutions	• Pour-flush toilets and water closets. • Countryman toilets (a term used in south-eastern Nigeria to refer to an improved pit latrine with a water closet squatting platform). • Ecological sanitation.
Description of good practices	The key activities implemented in the three states were: • community mobilization and sensitization, including meeting with traditional councils and community associations and entry processes on the project; • triggering using different participatory approaches; • developing commitment notes and action plans; • monitoring and follow-up activities; and • encouraging private entrepreneurs to stock hygiene and sanitation materials through the establishment of sanitation centres where community members could get further safe sanitation messages and buy materials for toilet construction.
Results	• More than 70% of the households in the small towns constructed latrines and are safely disposing of their faeces. • An average of about 40% of the households are practising effective handwashing. • Some artisans and entrepreneurs are selling sanitation materials and supporting latrine construction. • 400 communities achieved ODF status and are moving towards total sanitation.
Challenges	• The non-homogeneity of the people and elitist attitudes make community mobilization and management difficult in the small towns of Cross River State and Anambra. The involvement of Anambra State Association of Town Unions improved community engagement.

U-CLTS CASE STUDIES 163

- Informal settlement patterns and the land tenure system make it difficult to access land for latrine construction in Anambra East local government area (LGA).
- The toilet pits get filled up after a year or two due to the number of people using them. Emptying the pits is done manually and is usually expensive. For instance, in Bade LGA in Yobe, the average cost of emptying a pit is N20,000 (US$57). This often led to slippage when households could not afford the fee.
- There was weak sanitation chain management in Anambra, poor pit-emptying processes in Cross River, and unsafe treatment of human waste in Yobe.
- The settlement pattern and land tenure system make digging a new pit difficult, particularly in Anambra East LGA where there is little space and the soil type and riverine or flooding environment make this process problematic and expensive. In Fika LGA in Yobe, many full pits are abandoned due to the difficult topography and new latrines are constructed, with few reverting to OD.
- In Yobe, a sanitation centre was introduced in the CLTS implementation process as a pilot model (Abass and Dunia, 2009). The centre managers provide technical support for a minimal fee. Through this process, some households moved up the sanitation ladder.
- There are slippages with many small towns going back to OD due to latrine collapse, new people entering the community, and weak monitoring and follow-up.

Lessons
- The engagement and subsequent triggering of traditional, private, and governmental institutions in small towns led to rapid ODF and the construction of toilets. This was seen clearly in Cross River State.
- Inclusion of all ethnic groups and the introduction of Follow-up Mandona (FUM) in Cross River State and Benue provided a more focused and systematic process of supportive monitoring to ensure that communities committed to their promises.
- The establishment and training of Water Consumers' Associations (WCAs), adopting a positive deviance approach after achieving ODF, led to the identification of Natural Leaders who will support the sustainability of the CLTS programme. The functionality of the WCA in Cross River State is seen as being better than in Yobe and Anambra States.
- Segmentation of small towns into manageable CLTS areas means that they can be monitored easily.
- Sanitation marketing was integrated into the CLTS implementation process in Anambra. The involvement of private operators and entrepreneurs in running a business selling sanitation and hygiene materials (in Yobe State and through WaterAid in Jigawa) led to the upgrading of household and public toilets. This also reduced slippage.
- Institutional toilets were established in public places in Yobe (markets, motor parks, etc.). Allow for diverse solutions and approaches to toilets.

References Abass, K. and Dunia, E. (2009) 'Sanitation centre: a catalyst for the adoption of safe sanitation in small town, Yobe State, Nigeria', paper prepared for the West Africa Regional Sanitation and Hygiene Symposium, Accra, Ghana, 3–5 November, https://www.ircwash.org/resources/sanitation-centre-catalyst-adoption-safe-sanitation-small-town-yobe-state-nigeria-paper [accessed 25 February 2018].

http://wsssrp.org/anambra-state-working-to-end-open-defecation/ [accessed 25 February 2018].

www.wsssrp.org/Yobe [accessed 25 February 2018].

Conclusion

Achieving shit-free environments in all urban settings by 2030 is a complex challenge. It will require huge investments in institutional development, capacity building, and infrastructure combined with a repertoire of methods, tools, tactics, strategies, and approaches. U-CLTS could be an important piece of the puzzle. It has the potential to mobilize poor urban communities to take actions within their control and to collectively work with stakeholders to develop safely managed sanitation, hygiene, and water services. The tools outlined in this document create space for community participation in urban planning and management.

The aims of *Innovations for Urban Sanitation* are to:

- propose ways of integrating and adapting CLTS and other community-led strategies to different urban environments and to highlight the contribution they can make to different typologies; and
- stress the importance of:
  - adjusting to the local context;
  - working with other urban sanitation stakeholders;
  - considering the whole sanitation chain – containment, emptying, transportation, treatment, and reuse/disposal; and
  - embedding all sanitation initiatives into a larger town- or city-wide plan.

This guide has drawn on examples to provide guidance to those wishing to make urban sanitation more participatory and community-led. However, there are still many unknowns and areas that require further development and investigation.

The guide has avoided recommending a rigid structure for U-CLTS, and hopes to inspire adaptations and innovations. More work is needed to explore how the tools and tactics presented throughout the book can work with and strengthen existing mainstream approaches to networked and non-networked sanitation planning and implementation. We encourage readers to document and evaluate the work they undertake to share and improve knowledge and practice as well as to explore different ways in which CLTS approaches can be integrated into the provision of sustainable and equitable sanitation services across different urban typologies.

http://dx.doi.org/10.3362/9781780447360.007

Conclusion

References

Abass, K. and Dunia, E. (2009) 'Sanitation centre: a catalyst for the adoption of safe sanitation in small town, Yobe State, Nigeria', paper prepared for the West Africa Regional Sanitation and Hygiene Symposium, Accra, Ghana, 3–5 November. Available from: https://www.ircwash.org/resources/sanitation-centre-catalyst-adoption-safe-sanitation-small-town-yobe-state-nigeria-paper [accessed 25 February 2018].

Azafady (2015) *Adapting Rural CLTS for Urban Settings: Azafady UK's Experience in Fort-Dauphin, South East Madagascar*, Azafady, London. Available from: www.communityledtotalsanitation.org/sites/communityledtotalsanitation.org/files/Azafady_Adapting_rural_CLTS_for_urban_settings.pdf [accessed 7 November 2017].

Blackett, I. and Hawkins, P. (2017) *FSM Case Studies: Case Studies on the Business, Policy and Technology of Faecal Sludge Management*, 2nd edn, Bill and Melinda Gates Foundation, Seattle.

Blackett, I., Hawkins, P., and Heymans, C. (2014) 'The missing link in sanitation service delivery. A review of fecal sludge management in 12 cities', Water and Sanitation Programme (WSP) research brief, International Bank for Reconstruction and Development/World Bank, Washington DC.

BMGF (2015) *Building Demand for Sanitation. A 2015 Portfolio Update and Overview: Water, Sanitation, and Hygiene Strategy*, Bill and Melinda Gates Foundation (BMGF), Washington DC.

CARE Malawi (2013) *The Community Score Card (CSC): A Generic Guide for Implementing CARE's CSC Process to Improve Quality of Services*, CARE, Lilongwe. Available from: http://www.care.org/sites/default/files/documents/FP-2013-CARE_CommunityScoreCardToolkit.pdf [accessed 7 November 2017].

CCODE (2014) *Building Citywide Sanitation Strategies from the Bottom Up: A Situational Analysis for Blantyre City, Malawi*, SHARE Consortium, London. Available from: https://assets.publishing.service.gov.uk/media/57a089e2ed915d622c000447/SHAREResearchReport_Malawi_final.pdf [accessed 9 November 2017].

CESCR (2009) *General Comment No. 20 on Non-Discrimination*, UN Doc. E/C.12/GC/20, UN Committee on Economic, Social and Cultural Rights (CESCR), Geneva.

Chambers, R. (1983) *Rural Development: Putting the Last First*, Routledge, London.

Cole, B. (2013) 'Participatory design development for sanitation', *Frontiers of CLTS: Innovations and Insights* 1, Institute of Development Studies (IDS), Brighton. Available from: http://www.communityledtotalsanitation.org/sites/communityledtotalsanitation.org/files/media/Frontiers_of_CLTS_Issue1_PartDesign_0.pdf [accessed 22 February 2018].

Community-Led Total Sanitation Knowledge Hub (n.d.) [online]. Available from: www.communityledtotalsanitation.org [accessed 7 November 2017].

Coursera (no date) *Tools for Institutional and Political Economy Analysis for Sanitation Solutions* [online]. Available from: https://www.coursera.org/learn/sanitation/lecture/HyysG/5-6-tools-for-institutional-and-political-economy-analysis-for-sanitation [accessed 7 November 2017].

Dhu, B. (no date) *Challenges and Innovations of Urban Community-Led Total Sanitation: Case Study Findings from New Delhi, India*, unpublished report.

Ebener, S. (2008) *Training on Social Network Analysis, Mapping Social Relations*, World Health Organization, Manilla, Philippines. Available from: http://www1.paho.org/CDMEDIA/KMC-SNA/training-sna.htm [accessed 9 November 2017].

EY and WSUP (2017) *The World Can't Wait for Sewers*, Ernst and Young (EY) and Water and Sanitation for the Urban Poor (WSUP), London. Available from: http://www.ey.com/Publication/vwLUAssets/ey-the-world-cant-wait-for-sewers/$FILE/ey-the-world-cant-wait-for-sewers.pdf [accessed 9 November 2017].

Government of India (2018) *Swachh Survekshan 2018*, Ministry of Housing and Urban Affairs, Government of India, Delhi. Available from: https://swachhsurvekshan2018.org/Images/Swachh%20Survekshan%202018%20Toolkit%20-%20English.pdf [accessed 26 March 2018].

Government of Mozambique, Australian Aid, and UNICEF (2014) *NAMWASH Programme: Phase 1 Progress Report, January–December 2013*, unpublished report.

Guusu, S. and Chuktu, N. (no date) *Mob Triggering: An Urban CLTS Approach to Reaching Whole Clusters. The Experience of GSF-supported RUSHPIN Programme, Logo LGA, Benue State, Nigeria*, United Purpose, unpublished report.

Hanneman, R. and Riddle, M. (2005) *Introduction to Social Network Methods*, University of California, Riverside CA. Available from: http://www.faculty.ucr.edu/~hanneman/nettext/ [accessed 7 November 2017].

Hawkins P., Blackett I., and Heymans C. (2013) *Poor-inclusive Urban Sanitation: An Overview*, Water and Sanitation Programme (WSP), International Bank for Reconstruction and Development/World Bank, Washington DC. Available from: https://wedc-knowledge.lboro.ac.uk/resources/pubs/WSP-Poor-Inclusive-Urban-Sanitation-Overview.pdf [accessed 22 March 2018].

House, S., Ferron, S., and Cavill, S. (2017) 'Equality and non-discrimination (EQND) in sanitation programmes at scale', *Frontiers of CLTS* 10, Institute of Development Studies (IDS), Brighton. Available from: http://www.communityledtotalsanitation.org/sites/communityledtotalsanitation.org/files/Frontiers10_EQND.pdf [accessed 20 February 2018].

House, S., Ferron, S., Sommer, M., and Cavill, S. (2014) *Violence, Gender & WASH: A Practitioner's Toolkit – Making Water, Sanitation and Hygiene Safer through Improved Programming and Services*, 'Toolset 6: Violence experienced by people who may be vulnerable, marginalized or in special circumstances', WaterAid/SHARE, London.

Hueso, A. (2013) 'Sanitation in Nakuru's low-income urban areas', CLTS website blog [online]. Available from: http://www.communityledtotalsanitation.org/blog/sanitation-nakuru-s-low-income-urban-areas [accessed 25 February 2018].

ISF-UTS and SNV (2017) 'Exploring smart enforcement within urban sanitation', paper prepared by Chong, J., Murta, J., Kome, A., Grant, M., and

Willetts, J., Institute for Sustainable Futures, University of Technology, Sydney, for SNV Netherlands Development Organisation.

IUWASH (2015) *Improving Lifestyle and Health: A Guide to Urban Sanitation Promotion*, IUWASH, Jakarta. Available from: https://www.iuwashplus.or.id/cms/wp-content/uploads/2017/04/Guide-to-Urban-Sanitation-Promotion-EN.pdf [accessed 23 March 2018].

Jones, H. (2015) *Dialogue Circle on Social Inclusion: Guidance Note*, Water, Engineering and Development Centre (WEDC), Loughborough University, Loughborough. Available from: http://wedc.lboro.ac.uk/resources/learning/EI_Dialogue_circle_on_social_inclusion_guidance_note.pdf [accessed 9 November 2011].

Joshi, D. and Morgan, J. (2007) 'Pavement dwellers' sanitation activities: visible but ignored', *WaterLines* 25 (3): 19–22, DOI:10.3362/0262-8104.2007.007.

Kar, K. with Chambers, R. (2008) *Handbook on Community-Led Total Sanitation*, Plan International and Institute of Development Studies (IDS), London and Brighton. Available from: http://www.communityledtotalsanitation.org/resource/handbook-community-led-total-sanitation [accessed 23 February 2018].

Kar, K., Pradhan, S., Prabhakaran, P., Thomas, T., and Harvey, P. (forthcoming) *CLTS Rapid Appraisal Protocol (CRAP): A Tool for Rapid Assessment of the Practice of CLTS at Scale*, UNICEF and CLTS Foundation, New York and Kolkata.

Kooy, M. and Harris, D. (2012) *Political Economy Analysis for Water, Sanitation and Hygiene (WASH) Service Delivery*, Overseas Development Institute (ODI), London. Available from: https://www.odi.org/sites/odi.org.uk/files/odi-assets/publications-opinion-files/7797.pdf [accessed 7 November 2017].

Lundine, J., Kovačič, P., and Poggiali, L. (2012) 'Youth and digital mapping in urban informal settlements: lessons learned from participatory mapping processes in Mathare in Nairobi, Kenya', *Children, Youth and Environments* 22 (2): 214–33. Available from: https://www.researchgate.net/publication/259751234 [accessed 23 March 2018].

Lüthi, C., Morel, A., Tilley, E.. and Ulrich, L. (2011) *Community-Led Urban Environmental Sanitation: CLUES. A Complete Guide for Decision Makers with 30 Tools*, Eawag, UN-Habitat, and WSSCC, Dübendorf, Switzerland. Available from: http://www.eawag.ch/fileadmin/Domain1/Abteilungen/sandec/schwerpunkte/sesp/CLUES/CLUES_Guidelines.pdf [accessed 25 February 2018].

McHugh, K., Hountondji, J., Seiba, S., Zinsou, C., Kelly, G., and Poyer, S. (2015) *Efficiently Identifying and Addressing Market Failures in Urban Sanitation in West Africa*, poster presentation, UNC Water and Health Conference, Chapel Hill NC.

Mitlin, D. (2014) *Achieving Universal Sanitation: Sharing the Experience of the SDI Affiliate in Blantyre, Malawi*, International Institute for Environment and Development (IIED), London. Available from: https://www.iied.org/achieving-universal-sanitation-sharing-experience-sdi-affiliate-blantyre-malawi [accessed 9 November 2017].

Muller, M. and Beaver, K. (2013) *Water Supply, Sanitation and Hygiene in Nampula Province (NAMWASH), Mozambique*, evaluation report, Water and Development Management and Ipsos MORI. Available from: https://dfat.

gov.au/about-us/publications/Documents/mozambique-namwash-evaluation-2013.pdf [accessed 25 February 2018].

Musyoki, S. (2010) *Piloting CLTS in an Urban Setting: Diary of Progress in Mathare 10, Nairobi, Kenya*, blog [online]. Available from: http://www.communityledtotalsanitation.org/sites/communityledtotalsanitation.org/files/media/Mathare_blog_all.pdf [accessed 7 November 2017].

Myers, J. (2016) *Plan Netherlands' Experience of Using a CLTS Approach in Urban Environments*, Plan Nederland, Amsterdam. Available from: http://www.communityledtotalsanitation.org/sites/communityledtotalsanitation.org/files/Urban_CLTS_Plan.pdf [accessed 5 September 2016].

Myers, J., Pasteur, K., and Cavill, S. (2016) *The Addis Agreement: Using CLTS in Peri-urban and Urban Areas*, CLTS Knowledge Hub learning paper, Institute of Development Studies (IDS), Brighton. Available from: www.communityledtotalsanitation.org/sites/communityledtotalsanitation.org/files/The_Addis_Agreement_CLTS_urban_0.pdf [accessed 7 October 2017].

Nguyen, V., Nguyen-Viet, H., Pham-Duc, P., and Wiese, M. (2014) 'Scenario planning for community development in Vietnam: a new tool for integrated health approaches?', *Global Health Action* 7 (1): 10, http://doi:10.3402/gha.v7.24482 [accessed 23 February 2018].

Nique, M. and Smertnik, H. (2015) *Mobile for Development Utilities Programme: The Role of Mobile in Improved Sanitation Access*, GSMA, London. Available from: https://www.gsma.com/mobilefordevelopment/wp-content/uploads/2015/08/The-Role-of-Mobile-in-Improved-Sanitation-Access.pdf [accessed 9 November 2017].

ODI (2009) 'Political economy analysis: how to note', DFID practice paper, Overseas Development Institute (ODI), London. Available from: https://www.odi.org/sites/odi.org.uk/files/odi-assets/events-documents/3797.pdf [accessed 7 November 2017].

Pasteur, K. (2017) 'Keeping track: CLTS monitoring, certification and verification', CLTS Knowledge Hub learning paper, Institute of Development Studies (IDS), Brighton. Available from: http://www.communityledtotalsanitation.org/sites/communityledtotalsanitation.org/files/Keeping_Track_LearningPaper_0.pdf [accessed 22 February 2018].

Pasteur, K. and Prabhakaran, P. (2015) *Lessons in Urban Community-Led Total Sanitation from Nakuru, Kenya*, Practical Action, Rugby. Available from: www.communityledtotalsanitation.org/sites/communityledtotalsanitation.org/files/PracticalAction_LessonsOnUrbanCLTSNakuruKenya_Apr2015.pdf [accessed 7 October 2017].

Pasteur, K. and Prabhakaran, P. with Kar, K. (2016) *Achieving Open Defecation Free Gulariya Municipality*, CLTS Foundation, Kolkata. Available from: http://www.cltsfoundation.org/wp-content/uploads/2017/03/Gulariya-Municipality_Nepal_CLTS-Foundation_Practical-Action.pdf [accessed 9 November 2017].

Peal, A., Evans, B., Blackett, I., Hawkins, P., and Heymans, C. (2014) 'Fecal sludge management (FSM): analytical tools for assessing FSM in cities', *Journal of Water, Sanitation and Hygiene for Development* 4 (3): 371–83 https://doi.org/10.2166/washdev.2014.139 [accessed 23 February 2018].

Plan India (2014) *Urban Community-Led Total Sanitation in Delhi*, Plan India, New Delhi. Available from: http://www.communityledtotalsanitation.org/

sites/communityledtotalsanitation.org/files/media/UCLTS_Delhi_Report_Plan.pdf [accessed 7 November 2017].

Plan International, Because I am a Girl, Women in Cities International, and UN-Habitat (2013) *Adolescent Girls' Views on Safety in Cities: Findings of the Because I am a Girl Urban Programme Study in Cairo, Delhi, Hanoi, Kampala and Lima*, Plan International, Women in Cities International, and UN-Habitat, Woking, Montreal, and New York.

Practical Action (no date a) *Participatory Market System Development Roadmap*, Practical Action, Rugby. Available from: http://www.pmsdroadmap.org/ [accessed 7 November 2017].

Practical Action (no date b) *Total Sanitation in Nakuru Slums*, collation of project materials, video, blogs, papers, etc., Practical Action, Rugby. Available from: https://practicalaction.org/realising-the-right-to-total-sanitation-in-nakuru-slums [accessed 25 February 2018].

Quayle, T. (2012) 'UCLTS in Mathare 10, Nairobi', ACCESSanitation case study, ACCESSanitation, Nairobi. Available from: http://www.communityledtotalsanitation.org/resource/access-case-study-uclts-mathare-10-nairobi [accessed 25 February 2018].

Ross, I., Scott, R., Blackett, I.C., and Hawkins, P.M. (2016a) 'Fecal sludge management: diagnostics for service delivery in urban areas – summary report', Water and Sanitation Program technical paper, World Bank Group, Washington DC. Available from: http://documents.worldbank.org/curated/en/909691468338135561/Fecal-sludge-management-diagnostics-for-service-delivery-in-urban-areas-summary-report [accessed 22 February 2018].

Ross, I., Scott, R., Mujica, A., White, Z., and Smith, M. (2016b) 'Fecal sludge management: diagnostics for service delivery in urban areas – tools and guidelines', Water and Sanitation Program technical paper, World Bank Group, Washington DC. Available from: http://documents.worldbank.org/curated/en/461321468338637425/Fecal-sludge-management-diagnostics-for-service-delivery-in-urban-areas-tools-and-guidelines [accessed 22 February 2018].

SEED Madagascar (2017) *Final Report for Project Malio: A Community-led Approach to Eliminating OD and Facilitating Sustained Behaviour Change*, SEED Madagascar, London. Available from: https://madagascar.co.uk/application/files/8515/0461/2575/Project_Malio_Final_Report_July_2017.pdf [accessed 25 February 2018].

Shakya, H.B., Christakis, N.A., and Fowler, J.H. (2015) 'Social network predictors of latrine ownership', *Social Science and Medicine* 125: 129–38. Available from: http://fowler.ucsd.edu/social_network_predictors_of_latrine_ownership.pdf [accessed 22 February 2018].

Solomon, Y. (2013) *CLTS in Himbirti, Asmara, Eritrea*, UNICEF Eritrea, Asmara. Available from: http://www.communityledtotalsanitation.org/resource/achieving-odf-peri-urban-settings-clts-himbirti [accessed 25 February 2018].

SSWM (no date) *Venn Diagrams*, Sustainable Sanitation and Water Management [online]. Available from: https://www.sswm.info/content/venn-diagrams [accessed 9 November 2017].

Stevens, L. (2013) 'Realising the right to total sanitation: hybrid community-led total sanitation in Nakuru, Kenya', Practical Action blog [online].

Available from: https://practicalaction.org/blog/where-we-work/kenya/realising-the-right-to-total-sanitation-hybrid-clts-in-nakuru/ [accessed 25 February 2018].

Stevens, L., de la Brosse, N., and Casey, J. (2017) *Faecal Sludge Management and Technology Justice: Promoting Sustained and Scalable Solutions*, paper prepared for the 40th Water, Engineering and Development Centre (WEDC) International Conference, Loughborough University.

Stevens, L., Islam, R., Morcrette, A., de la Brosse, N., and al Mamun, A. (2015) *Faecal Sludge Management in Faridpur, Bangladesh: Scaling up through Service Level Agreements*, paper prepared for the 38th Water, Engineering and Development Centre (WEDC) International Conference, Loughborough University.

SuSanA (n.d.) *Shit Flow Diagrams*, Sustainable Sanitation Alliance [online]. Available from: www.sfd.susana.org/sfd [accessed 9 November 2017].

Thieme, T. (2010) 'Youth, waste and work in Mathare: whose business and whose politics?', *Environment and Urbanization* 22 (2): 333–52. Available from: http://journals.sagepub.com/doi/pdf/10.1177/0956247810379946 [accessed April 2018]

Thomas, A. and Alvestegui, A. (2015) 'Sanitation in small towns: experience from Mozambique', Eastern and Southern Africa Learning Series, UNICEF, Nairobi. Available from: www.unicef.org/esaro/WASH-Field-Small-Towns-low-res.pdf [accessed 9 November 2017].

Tilley, E., Ulrich, L., Lüthi, C., Reymond, P., and Zurbrügg, C. (2014) *Compendium of Sanitation Systems and Technologies*, Eawag, Dübendorf, Switzerland. Available from: http://www.eawag.ch/en/department/sandec/publications/compendium/ [accessed 4 January 2018].

UNICEF ESARO (2015) 'Real-time monitoring of rural sanitation at scale in Zambia using mobile to web technologies', WASH field note, UNICEF ESARO, Nairobi. Available from: https://www.unicef.org/esaro/WASH-Field-M2W-low-res.pdf [accessed 9 November 2017].

UNICEF Nigeria (2014) *Community-Led Total Sanitation in Nigeria: Case Studies*, UNICEF Nigeria, Abuja. Available from: http://www.communityledtotalsanitation.org/sites/communityledtotalsanitation.org/files/media/CLTS_Case_Studies_Nigeria.pdf [accessed 7 November 2017].

USAID and IUWASH (no date a) *Optimizing Coverage of Existing Master Meter and Triggering Community-based Total Sanitation in Sidoarjo District, East Java Province*, information sheet, USAID and Indonesia Urban Water, Sanitation, and Hygiene (IUWASH), Surabaya. Available from: https://www.iuwashplus.or.id/cms/wp-content/uploads/2017/04/Info-Sheet-Grants-in-Lemah-Putro-EN.pdf [accessed 25 February 2018].

USAID and IUWASH (no date b) *Program Profile: Community-based Total Sanitation Approach in Probolinggo City*, USAID and Indonesia Urban Water, Sanitation, and Hygiene (IUWASH), Surabaya. Available from: https://www.iuwashplus.or.id/cms/wp-content/uploads/2017/05/Program-Profile-STBM-in-Probolinggo-EN.pdf [accessed 25 February 2018].

Walnycki, A. and Schermbruker, N. (2016) *How Collective Action Strategies of the Urban Poor Can Improve Access to Sanitation*, SHARE Consortium, London. Available from: https://www.shareresearch.org/research/how-collective-action-strategies-urban-poor-can-improve-access-sanitation [accessed 7 November 2017].

WASH BAT (2016) *WASH Bottleneck Analysis Tool* [online]. Available from: http://www.washbat.org/ [accessed 7 November 2017].

WaterAid (2016) *A Tale of Clean Cities: Insights for Planning Urban Sanitation from Ghana, India and the Philippines*, synthesis and full reports, WaterAid, London.

WEDC (2017) *Equity and Inclusion in Water, Sanitation and Hygiene: Learning Materials*, Water, Engineering and Development Centre (WEDC), Loughborough University, Loughborough. Available from: https://wedc-knowledge.lboro.ac.uk/collections/equity-inclusion/general.html [accessed 7 November 2017].

WHO and UNICEF (2016) *Progress on Sanitation and Drinking Water: 2015 update and MDG Assessment*, World Health Organization (WHO)/UNICEF Joint Monitoring Programme, Geneva. Available from: http://files.unicef.org/publications/files/Progress_on_Sanitation_and_Drinking_Water_2015_Update_.pdf [accessed 9 November 2017].

WHO and UNICEF (2017) *Progress on Drinking Water, Sanitation and Hygiene: 2017 Update and SDG Baselines*, World Health Organization (WHO)/UNICEF Joint Monitoring Programme, Geneva. Available from: https://www.unicef.org/publications/files/Progress_on_Drinking_Water_Sanitation_and_Hygiene_2017.pdf [accessed 7 November 2017].

Wilbur, J. and Jones, H. (2014) 'Disability: making CLTS fully inclusive', *Frontiers of CLTS: Innovations and Insights* 3, Institute of Development Studies (IDS), Brighton. Available from: http://www.communityledtotalsanitation.org/sites/communityledtotalsanitation.org/files/Frontiers_of_CLTS_Issue3_Disabilities.pdf [accessed 22 February 2018].

Wild, L., Wales, J., and Chambers, V. (2015) *CARE's Experience with Community Score Cards: What Works and Why?*, Overseas Development Institute (ODI), London. Available from: https://www.odi.org/sites/odi.org.uk/files/odi-assets/publications-opinion-files/9451.pdf [accessed 7 November 2017].

Women in Cities International, Jagori, and International Development Research Centre (2011) *Gender and Essential Services in Low-income Communities. Report Findings of the Action Research Project: Women's Rights and Access to Water and Sanitation in Asian Cities*, Women in Cities International and Jagori, Montreal and Delhi.

World Vision Ethiopia (no date) *The Urban WASH Field Reports, August 2014–2017*, unpublished report.

WSP (2014) *Kenya State of Sanitation: Country Profiles*, Water and Sanitation Program (WSP) and World Bank, Washington DC. Available from: https://www.wsp.org/sites/wsp.org/files/publications/WSP-Kenya-47-County-Sanitation-Profiles-2014.pdf [accessed 9 November 2017].

WSUP (2014) *The Urban Programming Guide: How to Design and Implement an Effective Urban WASH Programme*, Water and Sanitation for the Urban Poor (WSUP), London. Available from: https://www.wsup.com/insights/the-urban-programming-guide-how-to-design-and-implement-an-effective-urban-wash-programme/ [accessed 9 November 2017].

WSUP (2016) 'Improving the quality of public toilet services in Kumasi', WSUP practice note, Water and Sanitation for the Urban Poor (WSUP), London. Available from: https://www.wsup.com/insights/improving-the-quality-of-public-toilets-in-kumasi/ [accessed 9 November 2017].

Yap, C. (2015) *Water and Sanitation Action Research in the City of Chinhoyi: Community Mapping Towards Inclusive Development*, SHARE Consortium, London. Available from: https://assets.publishing.service.gov.uk/media/57a089e540f0b649740002f8/Chinhoyi_Zimbabwe_POLICY_BRIEF.pdf [accessed 7 November 2017].

Zulu, G. (2011) *Urban CLTS in Zambia: The Case of Choma and Lusaka*, UNICEF Zambia, Lusaka. Available from: http://www.communityledtotalsanitation.org/resource/urban-clts-zambia [accessed 25 February 2018].

www.ingramcontent.com/pod-product-compliance
Ingram Content Group UK Ltd.
Pitfield, Milton Keynes, MK11 3LW, UK
UKHW021826140426
5217IPUK00004B/105